Isms

in Health Care Human Resources

A CONCISE GUIDE TO WORKPLACE DIVERSITY, EQUITY, AND INCLUSION

Darren Liu, DrPH, MHA, MS
Associate Professor, Des Moines University, Des Moines, Iowa

Betty Burston, PhD
Professor-in-residence, University of Nevada, Las Vegas, Las Vegas, Nevada

Shartriya Collier Stewart, MEd, EdD
Associate Dean, School of Education, Nevada State College, Las Vegas, Nevada

Heidi H. Mulligan
Owner, A Woman of A Thousand Words, Henderson, Nevada

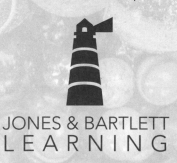

JONES & BARTLETT
LEARNING

World Headquarters
Jones & Bartlett Learning
5 Wall Street
Burlington, MA 01803
978-443-5000
info@jblearning.com
www.jblearning.com

Jones & Bartlett Learning books and products are available through most bookstores and online booksellers. To contact Jones & Bartlett Learning directly, call 800-832-0034, fax 978-443-8000, or visit our website, www.jblearning.com.

21975-3

Production Credits

VP, Product Management: Amanda Martin
Director of Product Management: Laura Pagluica
Product Manager: Sophie Fleck Teague
Content Strategist: Tess Sackmann
Manager, Project Management: Lori Mortimer
Senior Digital Project Specialist: Angela Dooley
Senior Marketing Manager: Susanne Walker
VP, Manufacturing and Inventory Control:
   Therese Connell

Composition: Exela Technologies
Project Management: Exela Technologies
Cover Design: Michael O'Donnell
Media Development Editor: Faith Brosnan
Rights Specialist: Maria Maimone
Cover Image (Title Page, Chapter Opener):
   © Rudmer Zwerver/Shutterstock
Printing and Binding: McNaughton & Gunn

Library of Congress Cataloging-in-Publication Data

Names: Liu, Darren, 1974- author. | Burston, Betty (Betty C.), author.
Title: Isms in health care human resources : a concise guide to workplace diversity, equity, and inclusion / Darren Liu, Betty Burston.
Description: Burlington, MA : Jones & Bartlett Learning, [2021] | Includes bibliographical references and index. | Summary: "The negative effects of ethnocentrism, genderism, and heterosexism in health care workplaces are underexplored. Additionally, conflicts within the workplace due to IQism – a bias against individuals with very high IQs – have not yet entered into public discussion. Yet, health care personnel, according to current research, is inclusive of large numbers of persons with IQs that place them within three standard deviations from the norms. These individuals often experience circumstances that constrain their output. Second, when various 'isms' are discussed in health care human resource management and/or health care management textbooks, the primary focus is compliance with current laws that forbid discrimination, as well as recommending cultural competency training for workers during the onboarding process or as part of the organization's employee development training. Third, health care human resources and/or health management textbooks bypass the complex trans-disciplinary variables which interact to generate and sustain the active operation of 'isms' in the workplace." – Provided by publisher.
Identifiers: LCCN 2020007647 | ISBN 9781284201802 (paperback)
Subjects: MESH: Attitude of Health Personnel | Cultural Competency | Prejudice–ethnology | Organizational Culture | Workplace | United States
Classification: LCC RA971.35 | NLM W 62 | DDC 362.1068/3–dc23
LC record available at https://lccn.loc.gov/2020007647

ISBN: 9781284201802

6048

Printed in the United States of America
24 23 22 21 20   10 9 8 7 6 5 4 3 2 1

Brief Contents

Contents

Preface

In your organization, do gifted employees or those who embody unique perspectives have high retention rates? Do you as a healthcare organization's leader always make top-down decisions although you lay claim to having incorporated a system of shared governance? Are the "voices" who make recommendations in your organization's meetings dominated by homogenous groups who have achieved "seniority" and who direct incivilities toward those who are "different"? If your answer is "yes" to any of these three questions, there may be subtle forces at work in your organization that constrain the maximization of output because of diversity.

"Diversity?" Your emotions whisper to your intellect.

"Diversity? I'm absolutely tired of hearing that term! My patience is exhausted by the efforts of our healthcare organization to achieve diversity, equity, and inclusion." Your emotions say to your cognitive apparatus!

"Every time I hear those terms, I'm overwhelmed with guilt!" Suddenly, you hear another voice saying to you,

"But, diversity and inclusion are not about accusations regarding the inequities." And then the voice continues….

Diversity references noticeable heterogeneity, variety, or multifariousness. A culture of diversity is one that welcomes different perspectives from others without regard to their race/ethnicity, age, sex, seniority and/or other isms such as those discussed in this book. Organizations that truly value diversity, equity, and inclusion will seek to help maximize outcomes across their diverse workplaces. Whether one is born a leader, or has learned to lead, healthcare administrators are called upon to shape a culture that utilizes diversity, equity, and inclusion as opportunities to deliver the maximum possible levels of goods or services. This book was written to facilitate this process by using lessons from the past to inform the future.

In learning lessons from the past, differences are often more valuable than similarities. During each period of human existence, humankind has faced threats to its continued survival. During each key era, the survival of homo sapiens has been contingent upon the type of tools conceived and created, and the nature and the organization of the human systems that were designed to support survival. As Earth's residents move toward its undisclosed future, it is these same sets of resources that will interactively allow its inhabitants to successfully protect itself from the gamma ray bursts that accompany the "deaths" of galaxies and/or other threats. Thus, the maximization of output by every single person is integral to the continuation of that species of life which we call humans. More concretely, every single organization must create conditions that allow their workers to use their various gifts and talents to deliver the maximum possible levels of goods and services.

Yet, very few workplaces engage in output maximization so that humankind can advance and strengthen the planet's survival resources. Rather, micro-level conflicts and responses to these conflicts, intergroup squabbling and bickering, in-group/out-group accusations, and other such interactions subtract from human-kind's possibilities and probabilities at the very point in history when the potential-ities laid dormant or terminally injured from such behaviors generate losses that we cannot afford.

At the time of the writing of this preface, the global population was undergo-ing a tremendous challenge in human history—the Coronavirus (COVID-19) out-break, a deadly respiratory illness that had infected more than 8 millions people and claimed the lives of more than 435,000 people (WHO, 2020). In the United States, there were more than 2.1 million confirmed cases and over 117,000 deaths. This crisis provides historical proof of the need for humans to act in oneness and not in divisiveness. During the COVID-19 pandemic, organizations and countries practicing diversity and operating within the framework of the inclusive leadership were able to respond more quickly (Wang, Ng & Brook, 2020). Leadership, in this case, was not based on social justice. Rather, it required the maximization of output by healthcare administrators and other healthcare professionals.

Simultaneously, events also occurred in the United States that revealed the continuity of incivilities based on the "Ism" called Race. A specific event catalyzed the re-energization of the Black Lives Matter movement in the country. Protests and marches took place not only in the United States, but in countries across the globe. These demonstrations, in some cases, resulted in adverse events such as looting, destruction of property, injuries, and even death. Moreover, due to these events occurring during the worldwide pandemic, while not yet fully substantiated, COVID-19 cases are predicted to rise given the lack of social distancing during these large gatherings. These events have left those who value the gift that each human is to each other bewildered, saddened, and, in many cases, hopeless that human dif-ferences will continue to be assigned designations of inferiority and/or superiority and subjected to all manners of incivilities as a result of such beliefs, attitudes, and related behaviors.

Yet, the coalescence of a biological pandemic and a highly visible one based upon the intersectionality of RACE-ISM, CLASS-ISM, NATION-ISM, POLITICAL-ISM, and an array of other "Isms," has demonstrated an indisputable point—that "Isms" across categories support an exponential increase in incivilities and it is these resulting incivilities that compromise the unity needed for the collective survival of humankind. While this book focuses upon the impact of "Isms" in healthcare workplaces, it provides a framework that informs us that "Isms" cannot be singularly added. The commitment to diminish and ultimately eliminate that "Ism" called race, in order to be successful, requires humans to introspect, identify the various "Isms" that reside within their own spirits, bodies, and minds, and to evict them.

Humans must also be willing to work together as a collective to ensure the worldwide elimination of these "Isms." The change that has been in-waiting since humans migrated from the cradle of their beginning on a land-mass now known as Africa requires that humankind rise as a collective and say, "Yes, we are differ-ent, but we, as humankind, are made better by our differences and every single one of us pledge to no longer elevate and/or denigrate as a result of these differences." Whether our incivility towards another remains lodged in an unburied region of our brain and/or in power achieved by resources and/or social position, we will not direct incivilities borne of adverse beliefs, attitudes, or behaviors towards each other." It is interesting that some of the same strategies that can reduce the operation of "Isms" in healthcare workplaces can also reduce the health risks that occur as a result of "Isms" in other arenas of life. When analyzed, the content matter of this text provides tips for how we, as caring humans, can diminish and/or reduce "Isms" to a level of statistical and operative insignificance.

The purpose of this book is that of introducing an alternative framework for re-analyzing ways to reverse the operation of "Isms" in healthcare workplaces. Specifically, we assess the impact of negative attitudes and beliefs about groups of individuals who embody characteristics that differ from the "norm" for our society. We apply the term, "Isms" to such beliefs and behaviors. These various "Isms" are of such a magnitude that overall workplace productivity is diminished by their presence. While many "Isms" exist, we have chosen to specifically discuss sexualisms, IQism, heterosexism, and cultural diversitisms. However, one goal of this book is that of providing an easy-to-read tool that can accompany undergraduate and/or graduate textbooks in Public Health Leadership, Healthcare Administration & Management, and/or Human Resources Management courses. But, the ultimate objective of this book is that of motivating humans to explore the "Isms" which they embody, and to commit to no longer engaging in the incivilities which we often direct towards others because of our "Isms."

Chapter 1 presents the background and defines the concept of diversity in the healthcare workforce. We begin with a description of the demographic composition of the healthcare workforce by race/ethnicity and gender. (These data were taken from the U.S. Department of Labor, Bureau of Labor Statistics.) In addition, we also introduce several commonly held "Isms" and discuss how they may operate in healthcare workplaces. We then conclude that in order to "maximize" workplace outcomes, managers and administrators must behave strategically in hiring, building, leading, and managing their teams.

This text is based on the framework of the *Theory of Central Tendencyism*—a theory that we conceptualized from a statistical concept. Chapter 2 explains why some people respond to various individuals and groups in the workplace through behavioral incivilities. The overall goal for the learners is to recognize and avoid "uncivil" behaviors via self-reflection on the underdeveloped humanisms that accompany "Isms" when such behaviors appear in workplaces.

Chapter 3 specifically focuses on sexualisms and propinquity in healthcare workplaces as a framework for understanding sexual harassment, sexual assault, and related incivilities. In order to delineate the negative relationship between sexualism and outcome maximization, we introduce Title VII of the Civil Rights Act of 1964 and Equal Employment Opportunity Commission (EEOC). Data are presented on what has happened in the past to selected healthcare organizations that have failed to comply with the regulations. Several original solutions are also provided to guide healthcare administrators in addressing these issues.

Chapter 4 introduces the concept of IQism and documents its operation within healthcare and other workplaces. The discussions is then expanded by identifying ways that people with extraordinary cognitive skills can be better managed so that output is maximized. Throughout this chapter, however, the benefits of blending the optimal mix of "intelligences" is emphasized.

Chapter 5 discusses an often-missing component in the overall portrait of healthcare workforce diversity by discussing the operation of heterosexism—yet another "Ism" that can impede output maximization in a healthcare or other workplace. This chapter documents the increase in the number and percent of sexual minorities in the workplace. Strategies for addressing heterosexism to support the output maximization are outlined in detail.

Chapter 6 summarizes the "Isms" that are discussed in the first five chapters and introduces additional strategies for reducing "Isms" as barriers in healthcare and other workplaces. This chapter begins by reviewing a sample of recent Equal Employment Opportunity Commission (EEOC) cases involving healthcare workplaces. Chapter 6 concludes with recommendations for behavioral change strategies to ensure that employees self-analyze and confront their own attitudes and behaviors toward the goal of supporting a workplace characterized by cooperation and accommodation.

Finally, Chapter 7 consists of an epilogue suggesting that each of us, as healthcare workers, must constantly ask the question, *"Did I apply civilities in every area of my gross and nuanced behavior today?"*

Given the scarcity of educational materials in this area, we humbly introduce this book in the hope that the current and future senior-level public health and healthcare administrators/managers will read, reflect on the contents, and, most importantly, implement some of the productivity-enhancing strategies that are suggested. But, we are also hopeful that these brief comments will support our primary purpose—building on an existent body of transdisciplinary research to support active change in healthcare and other workplaces. We are extremely grateful to our long-time friend and colleague, Kurt Houser, FACHE. Despite his position as the Chief Human Resources Officer at one of the largest hospitals in Las Vegas, Nevada, he provided an unbiased review and valuable feedback in terms of the potential value of this book to healthcare managers and human resources personnel. Equally important, we would like to thank the team of Senior Managers from Jones & Bartlett Learning who welcomed and encouraged our highly unique approaches on a prior text, *The Challenges of Health Disparities: Implications and Actions for Health Care Professionals* (Liu et al., 2019), and once again on this "Isms" book. For this, we are most grateful for our views on these issues that do, indeed, comprise a completely different perspective.

Darren Liu
Betty Burston
Heidi H. Mulligan
Shartriya Collier Stewart
June 15, 2020

References

Liu, D., Burston, B., Collier-Stewart, S., & Mulligan, H. H. (2019). *The Challenges of Health Disparities: Implications and Actions for Health Care Professionals*. Jones & Bartlett Learning.

Wang, C. J., Ng, C. Y., & Brook, R. H. (2020). Response to COVID-19 in Taiwan: Big data analytics, new technology, and proactive testing. *JAMA, 323*(14), 1341–1342. doi:10.1001/jama.2020.3151

World Health Organization. Coronavirus Disease (2019). Coronavirus disease (COVID-19) Situation Report – 147. https://www.who.int/emergencies/diseases/novel-coronavirus-2019/situation-reports

Foreword

After 80 plus years, Dale Carnegie's (1937) advice seems to still be valid! In his classic book, *How to Win Friends and Influence People*, he argued that a person's financial success is determined more by the ability to "deal with people" than by "technical knowledge." More recent studies by the Carnegie Institute of Technology revealed that 85% of financial success is due to skills in "human engineering," or one's ability to communicate, function in a teamwork environment, and lead, while only 15% is due to technical knowledge. Nevertheless, our educational institutions disproportionately focus on technical and hard skill development. Continuing education in health care is also heavily centered on developing hard skills. In fact, I have heard senior leaders categorize the soft skills of communicating well, leading effectively, and building effective teams as "wasted efforts."

In his article, "The Neuroscience of Trust" in the *Harvard Business Review*, Paul Zak (2017) argues that a "soft skill" such as creating a culture of trust results in the stimulation of *oxytocin*. The release of this chemical results in increased trust and "reduces the fear of trusting a stranger." His findings conclude that organizations and leaders can produce a natural competitive advantage by hiring and developing leaders who are trustworthy, leaders whose followers trust them to treat them fairly and equitably. Zak demonstrates that trust in the leader results in lower turnover, higher employee engagement, greater productivity, fewer sick days, and several other measures of effectiveness that a CEO or HR chief would greatly welcome. These so-called soft skills are vital in today's competitive environment for recruiting and retaining high-quality healthcare talent. The changing population demographics, the increasing knowledge of our patient base, and the need for culturally competent leaders in all areas of healthcare call for leaders who know how to build, motivate, and retain a diverse team of persons who are, themselves, talented leaders.

Yet, to achieve these outcomes, workplaces need to take different approaches. Hiring for "cultural fit" has even gotten a bad rap these days. That's because the assumption of "cultural fit" embodies the premise that one must hire people who look, think, behave, and lead like you, the hiring manager, or the senior leader. In a seasoned organization, with a seasoned leader, this assumption is incorrect. In fact, when it comes to "cultural fit" for a mature leader who really wants a competitive advantage in his or her workplace, the opposite may be true. He or she must be open to hiring people unlike him or herself. He or she may choose to hire someone whose skills compensate for the leader's weaknesses, who thinks differently from the leader, and who will challenge the leader's decision-making for the betterment of the organization. Of course, this leader must not be insecure, must not be afraid to be challenged intellectually, and must not be vulnerable to his or her peers and/ or subordinates. Only then will the person truly have a diverse organization, one that is diverse not only in race, age, and sex but also in experiences, thoughts, and organizational personality.

Generally, the most impressive leaders have the most basic, but vital, soft skills. They know themselves. They understand their personality biases, either through assessments, such as DiSC (Scullard & Baum, 2015), Myers-Briggs Type Indicator (Quenk, 2009), or other tools that allow them to better understand themselves. This is the key takeaway from *Isms in Health Care Human Resources: A Concise Guide to Workplace Diversity, Equity, and Inclusion*. Through the numerous provided examples of "Isms," the authors demonstrate that the only way to affirmatively address them is by the leader first knowing, questioning, and improving him or herself through self-reflection. This is what will lead to authentic positive change among leaders, teams, and organizations as a whole. This book will cause every single healthcare manager and/or administrator to rethink the dynamics of human interaction in his or her workplace. This is a book that every current and future healthcare professional should read!

Kurt J. Houser, MBA, MS, FACHE
Chief, Human Resources Officer
University Medical Center of Southern Nevada
Las Vegas, Nevada

References

Carnegie, D. (1937). *How to Win Friends and Influence People*. New York: Simon and Schuster.
Quenk, N. L. (2009). *Essentials of Myers-Briggs Type Indicator Assessment*. John Wiley & Sons.
Scullard, M., & Baum, D. (2015). *Everything DiSC Manual*. John Wiley & Sons.
Zak, P. J. (2017). The neuroscience of trust. *Harvard Business Review, 95*(1), 84–90.

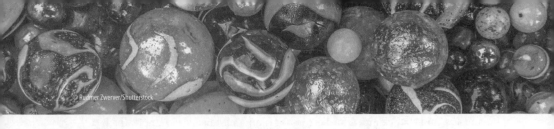

CHAPTER 1

Isms in Healthcare and Other Workplaces: An Overview

"A lot of different flowers make a bouquet."

– Muslim quote

LEARNING OBJECTIVES

After completing this chapter, each reader will be able to:

- Define the concept of "Ism" and identify key "Isms" that are observable in health care and other workplaces.
- Summarize data on the size and composition of the healthcare marketplace.
- Analyze and evaluate the limitations of viewing diversity in the healthcare workforce based only on race/ethnicity and/or gender.
- Craft and recommend strategies to further strengthen collaborative, cooperative, high-performing workplaces with diverse cultural groups in healthcare environments.

▶ Introduction: An Overview of the Demographic Composition in Healthcare Workplaces

Given the heterogeneity of the U.S. population, it is not surprising that healthcare workplaces are staffed by workers from diverse backgrounds.

With a population of over 330 million people (U.S. Bureau of the Census U.S. and World Population Clock, 2020), the United States is the third most populated country in the world. U.S. healthcare organizations willingly consent to serve its residents via their roles as employees, owners, consultants, and/or other participants in the healthcare system. Thus, healthcare institutions and their administrators, managers, and staff cannot afford errors for many reasons. For example, the health-care industry is constantly under scrutiny by individuals and other organizational entities. Martin Makary and Michael Daniel's well-known study (2016) explains the reason for such vigilance. The two authors suggest that the output of people in the healthcare industry includes errors that place healthcare professionals in the position of being the third cause of death in the United States (Makary and Daniel, 2016). Similarly, health care now employs a plurality of all workers within the U.S. economy. Additionally, the centrality of health care in day-to-day life has placed this unique institution at the center of policy debates.

Like the U.S. labor market in general, some analysts claim that healthcare organizations intentionally and/or unintentionally hire, manage, develop, pro-mote, and terminate workers based on criteria that extend beyond those related to actual and/or prospective performance. Acholonu et al. (2019) cited a 2018 report by the National Academies of Science, Engineering, and Medicine. This study revealed that while sexual harassment is culturally embedded within all sci-ence, technology, engineering, and mathematics (STEM) and related fields, these negative behaviors are most dominant in medicine. Coombs and King (2005) reported blatant discrimination in terms of job advancement, hiring, and other areas based on race/ethnicity, sex, international birth status, and other factors in healthcare workplaces 15 years ago. In 2013, the American Hospital Associ-ation's Institute for Diversity in Health Management (2014) found that racial/ethnic asymmetries existed in hospitals between the patients and the middle and senior-level executives who were the leaders and managers of these institutions.

Specifically, the American Hospital Association's Institute for Diversity exam-ined data that revealed an interesting pattern. While 31% of patients served were not of European descent, culturally concordant staff were severely underrepresented among the hospital administrators. Although racial/ethnic minorities accounted for 31% of patients, they were only 14% of Hospital Board members. That is, the proportion of patients who were minority was 121.4% greater than the percent of Board members who were minority. Similarly, minorities were only 12% of the total hospital executives. Thus, there were 158.3% more racial/minority patients than racial/minority hospital executives. Such data generate the need to more broadly examine the racial/ethnic and gender composition of the human resource pool of talent who collectively deliver health care within the United States.

Considering the lag, verification, and analysis of data on the national compo-sition of the health care and overall labor market, data from 2017 and 2018 were examined in 2020 (U.S. Department of Labor, 2017; U.S. Department of Labor 2018). In 2017, approximately 153,337,000 people aged 16 and older were working in the United States. In 2018, the number of workers had increased to approximately 155,761,000. Approximately 21,133,000 or 13.56% of these employees worked in health care. When the healthcare marketplace is disaggregated by type of job, race/ethnicity, and gender, a number of patterns emerge. For example, the medical and health service managers, sector experienced an aggregate decrease in the partic-ipation of African, Asian, and Latinx Americans. In contrast, in the healthcare practitioners and technical occupations sectors, participation increased for all races/ethnicities except Caucasian Americans. **TABLE 1.1** summarizes this data.

TABLE 1.1 Demography of Healthcare and Social Assistance Workers Versus All Workers, 2018

Industry	Total Number of Employees	% Women	% White Americans (including Latinx/Hispanics)	% African Americans	% Asian Americans	% Latinx/Hispanic Americans Only
Total Workers Age of 16 Years and Older in the American Workplace	155,761,000	46.9	78.0	12.3	6.3	17.3
Hospitals (33.99%) of all Healthcare Workers	7,108,000	75.0	73.1	15.4	8.9	10.9
Health Services, Except Hospitals (50.00% of all healthcare workers)	10,636,000	78.7	71.9	18.4	6.6	13.8
- Office of Physicians (15.0% of all nonhospital workers)	1,595,000	77.3	78.9	10.9	7.1	14.1
- Offices of Dentists (8.21% of all nonhospital workers)	873,000	84.0	83.9	5.8	6.9	18.7

(continues)

TABLE 1.1 Demography of Healthcare and Social Assistance Workers Versus All Workers, 2018   *(continued)*

Industry	Total Number of Employees	% Women	% White Americans (including Latinx/ Hispanics)	% African Americans	% Asian Americans	% Latinx/Hispanic Americans Only
- Offices of Chiropractors (1.36% of all nonhospital workers)	145,000	58.6	89.5	5.3	3.1	8.7
- Offices of Optometrists (1.5% of all nonhospital workers)	159,000	75.2	80.8	5.5	7.4	10.9
- Offices of Other Health Practices (3.34% of all nonhospital workers)	355,000	79.0	84.3	7.4	6.7	8.2
- Outpatient Care Centers (17.90% of all nonhospital workers)	1,904,000	76.7	76.2	14.6	6.2	14.0
- Home Healthcare Services (13.84% of all nonhospital workers)	1,472,000	87.9	63.0	26.1	7.2	18.5
- Other Healthcare Services (14.57% of all nonhospital workers)	1,550,000	70.2	68.0	20.0	9.1	12.0

Industry Nursing Care Facilities (Skilled Nursing Facilities) (15.53% of all healthcare and social assistance living providers)	1,652,000	84.2	63.5	28.3	5.6	11.0
Residential Care Facilities (Except Skilled Nursing Facilities) (8.7% of all healthcare and social assistance living workers)	930,000	74.3	66.6	26.3	3.9	12.2
Social Assistance (16.02% of all healthcare and social assistance living workers)	3,389,000	84.2	71.8	19.5	4.8	18.6
- Individual and Family Services (47.44% of all social assistance workers)	1,608,000	77.9	69.6	20.8	5.4	16.5
- Community Food and Housing and Emergency Services (3.69% of all social assistance workers)	125,000	67.3	74.2	19.7	1.7	15.0

(continues)

TABLE 1.1 Demography of Healthcare and Social Assistance Workers Versus All Workers, 2018 *(continued)*

Industry	Total Number of Employees	% Women	% White Americans (including Latinx/Hispanics)	% African Americans	% Asian Americans	% Latinx/Hispanic Americans Only
- Vocational Rehabilitation Services (2.77% of all social service workers)	94,000	54.5	71.4	24.3	0.3	15.6
- Child Day Care Services (46.73% of all social service workers)	1,562,000	93.8	73.8	18.1	4.7	21.2
Medical and Health Services Managers[a]	639,000	72.0	80.9	11.5	5.0	9.0
Healthcare Practitioners and Technical Occupations[a]	9,420,000	75.0	75.2	12.6	9.9	8.5
Healthcare and Social Assistance Workers[a]	21,133,000	78.4	72.3	17.5	7.1	13.6

Data from U.S. Department of Labor, Bureau of Labor Statistics, 2018, at Table 18. Employed persons by detailed industry, sex, race, and Hispanic or Latino ethnicity at https://www.bls.gov/cps/cpsaat18.pdf; [a]U.S. Department of Labor, Bureau of Labor Statistics, 2018, at Table 11. Employed persons by detailed occupation, sex, race, and Hispanic or Latino ethnicity at https://www.bls.gov/cps/cpsaat11.pdf

Table 1.1 includes the distribution of healthcare workers by sex, race/ethnicity, and the specific type of healthcare workplace in 2018.

When the data in Table 1.1 are comparatively analyzed, unique patterns are revealed that suggest exploring the racial/ethnic and sex distributional patterns in healthcare labor markets versus the patterns that are observable in the aggregate American economy. **BOX 1.1** lists a few of these trends.

The meaning of the data in Box 1.1 are clear. In a review of Ruth Milkman's newest book, *On Gender, Labor and Inequality*, Christina Gringeri (2019) highlights the fact that despite the rapid progress of equality in the American labor market that has occurred over recent decades, asymmetrical outcomes between male and female labor force participants can be documented. Thus, the statistically significant "surplus" of females in health care and health-related workplaces raises the question, "Are healthcare workplaces allowing total output to be negatively influenced by adverse gender-related beliefs, attitudes, and behaviors"?

Further research reveals that such a query is not only applicable to healthcare workplaces in the United States, but to healthcare workplaces at a global level. For example, Rubery (2019) documents differential treatment of healthcare workers by sex in Europe. Addabbo (2020) statistically assessed wage differences between male and female workers in European countries. Hsu and Lawler (2019) discuss mechanisms in the Taiwanese labor markets that may be related to decreased output maximization due to lack of gender diversity especially as it pertains to jobs at higher levels of complexity. Thus, across global healthcare marketplaces, gender interacts with race/ethnicity and other discriminators to form obstacles to output maximization (Maroto et al. 2019).

As Table 1.1 reveals, the racial/ethnic distribution of healthcare workplaces also differs from the patterns found in the United States in general. **BOX 1.2** identifies a few of these patterns.

Such distributions by race/ethnicity raise the question of whether such patterns have an impact on output maximization in healthcare workplaces. Some evidence suggests that race/ethnicity may affect output maximization. For example, the 2017 report, *Discrimination in America: Experiences and Views of Asian Americans* (Robert Wood Johnson Foundation, November 2017), found that 32% of Asians had experienced general discrimination, and 27% had experienced prejudice based on their ethnicity when applying for a job. Additionally, 25% had experienced discrimination in pay and promotions. Again, such findings raise the question, "Are such behaviors also operative in healthcare workplaces"?

▶ Beyond Race/Ethnicity and Gender

Ageism

The intersectionalities in the U.S. workplace go far beyond race/ethnicity and gender. Dennis and Thomas (2007) identified how beliefs and attitudes toward older people's productivity potential can be observed in workplaces such as "…media, healthcare, education, and advertising." Robert N. Butler (1969) introduced the term, "ageism", a concept that has since been redefined as applying

BOX 1.1 Gender Distribution Differences (American Healthcare Marketplaces Versus Other Labor Markets in General)

- Females are significantly over-represented in every single segment of the healthcare workplace.
  - For example, females are 46.9% of the overall workplace but 78.4% of all healthcare and social service workers.
  - When the percentage difference is calculated, we see that females are 67.16% more likely to work in health care than in the American economy as a whole.
- The following trends are revealed when the workplaces are disaggregated:
  - Females are 59.914% over-represented in hospitals.
  - When hospitals are excluded, females are 67.803% more likely to work in health service workplaces.
  - Females are 64.819% more likely to work in physicians' offices than they are to work in the overall economy.
  - Females are 79.10% more likely to work in Dentists' offices than they are to work in the overall economy.
  - While only 58.6% of all nonhospital workers who work for chiropractors are female, this percentage is 24.94% higher than the overall percentage of women in the workforce in general.
  - Approximately 75.2% of all persons employed by optometrists are females—a proportion that is 60.34% higher than for the overall economy.
  - The workplaces of home health services healthcare institutions are 87.9% female, a proportion that exceeds the overall economy by 87.42%.
  - Women are 70.2% of the employees in other healthcare services workplaces—an amount that is 49.68% greater than the proportion of women in the workplace in general.
  - Approximately 84.2% of all people who work in social assistance positions are female. This is 79.53% higher than the number of women in the overall workplace.
- When Social Assistance Workers are disaggregated into key occupations, other variables are also observable.
  - Approximately 77.9% of workers who deliver Individual and Family Services are female. Thus, there are 66.09% more females working in Individual and Family Services than there are females in the workplace in general.
  - Women are 66.5% of all Community Food and Housing and Emergency Services workers. This equates to 41.79% more women working in these unique healthcare workplaces than the percent of women who are employed in the overall workplace.
  - In Vocational Rehabilitation, 54.5% of all workers are women. Thus, only 16.204% more females are employed in this field than the percentage of women who are in the general workforce.
  - Finally, Child Day Care Service workers are 93.8% females. Thus, females are 100% more likely to work in child daycare services than their female counterparts in the general workplace.

Data from U.S. Department of Labor, Bureau of Labor Statistics, 2018, at Table 18. Employed persons by detailed industry, sex, race, and Hispanic or Latino ethnicity at https://www.bls.gov/cps/cpsaat18.pdf; U.S. Department of Labor, Bureau of Labor Statistics, 2018, at Table 11. Employed persons by detailed occupation, sex, race, and Hispanic or Latino ethnicity at https://www.bls.gov/cps/cpsaat11.pdf

BOX 1.2   Racial/Ethnic Distribution Differences (The American Healthcare Marketplaces Versus Other Labor Markets in General)

- Approximately 78.0% of all workers in the U.S. labor markets are classified as White Americans when Latinx Americans are included. The data in Column 3 of Table 1.1. reveal that:
  - People classified as White Americans are employed at rates that exceed their numbers in the overall economy for chiropractors (89.5%), optometrists (86.9%), dentists (83.9%), physicians (80.8%), and other health practitioners (84.3%).
  - In contrast, White Americans are under-represented in home healthcare services (63.0%), other healthcare services (68.0%), skilled nursing care facilities (63.5%), residential care facilities except skilled nursing facilities (66.6%), and in all social assistance workplaces (71.8%).
- When Latinx Americans are analyzed separately, they are 17.3% of all workplaces but only 13.6% of all healthcare and social assistance workers. Thus, on average, they are under-represented in this category of healthcare workers by 78.61%.
  - Latinx Americans are 18.6% of all social assistance workplaces. Thus, they are only over-represented by 7.514% in this unique health-related marketplace.
- In contrast, African Americans represent 12.3% of workers in the economy as a whole.
  - However, this group is over-represented by 42.28% among healthcare and social assistance workers.
  - Among physicians (10.9%), dentists (5.8%), chiropractors (5.3%), optometrists (5.5%), and other health practice offices (7.4%), this group is underrepresented.

Data from U.S. Department of Labor, Bureau of Labor Statistics, 2018, at Table 18. Employed persons by detailed industry, sex, race, and Hispanic or Latino ethnicity at https://www.bls.gov/cps/cpsaat18.pdf; U.S. Department of Labor, Bureau of Labor Statistics, 2018, at Table 11. Employed persons by detailed occupation, sex, race, and Hispanic or Latino ethnicity at https://www.bls.gov/cps/cpsaat11.pdf

preconceived beliefs about individuals that discount their worth based on their age (Achenbaum, 2014). While Wyman et al. (2018) focus upon **ageism** as it applies to bias against patients, ageism may also operate as a healthcare management or human resources management problem in healthcare workplaces. Fasbender et al. (2016) used a sample of 102 human resource management workers from multiple industries in the United States and identified beliefs and practices that involved unfair negative assessments of the contributions of older workers within their workplaces and, as a result, a lower willingness to hire older workers who sought employment opportunities. In a qualitative research study based on a sample of 28 older nurses, Rosenfeld (2007), for example, found that despite the nursing shortage, healthcare managers, together with the human resources department, did not attempt to retain older nurses. However, ageism needs more investigation in healthcare workplaces since it is an intersectionality that can interact with female and/or racial/ethnic status. Kydd and Fleming (2015) also sought to identify whether ageism is a set of beliefs, attitudes, and behaviors that are observable within healthcare workplaces.

In 2018, 16,911 age discrimination cases were filed with the Equal Employment Opportunity Commission (EEOC, 2018). One of these was filed against a Colorado Hospital (EEOC Press Release, 2018). The hospital had either terminated or coerced into resignation 29 employees who were aged 40 and over. Hospital personnel also made inappropriate age-related comments. The hospital agreed to pay $400,000 during settlement proceedings and to strengthen its anti-discrimination policy and trainings.

Lookism

Beliefs, assumptions, and behaviors regarding workers in healthcare and other workplaces can also occur because of a person's physical appearance. Symons (June 2, 2018) discusses a set of beliefs, attitudes, and behaviors based on physical appearance. Such reactions are called "lookism." While **lookism** has not been prohibited by legislation, Symons argues that when investigated by people whose area of training is bioethics, lookism is an exceptionally common phenomenon. Symons cites data from different sources. This data suggest that lookism is vast and can replicate and/or possibly exceed the magnitude of discrimination that is based on race/ethnicity, age, and/or religion.

Lee et al. (2017) argue that lookism can also have a very negative impact on overall health. Using long-term data based on a study of individuals from age 15 to 24 years of age, persons who were considered less attractive had worse health outcomes by the age of 24 years than the "more attractive" people who had earned higher social ratings. Warhurst et al. (2015) cite examples of lookism. These incidents ranged from physical appearance serving as a basis for admission into the Navy in China, to being hired as a stylist in a labor market in Glasgow, to the overall hiring processes in other industries and countries. The evidence revealed behavioral patterns that advantaged and/or disadvantaged workers based on physical appearance.

Lookism is not merely based on innate physical traits from birth. It also includes physical conditions that are directly and/or indirectly related to behavior. Lee et al. (2019) analyzed data on approximately 400 high school seniors and 2,000 students from middle schools included in the Korean Education and Employment Panel. The conclusion was that, in Korea, overweight and/or obese males experienced advantages in key types of jobs and wages relative to applicants of normal weight. In contrast, obese and overweight females were less likely to be hired. However, when hired, obese and/or overweight females were more likely to receive lower wages.

Pingitore et al. (1994) held facial "beauty" and other confounding factors constant by using 320 of the same males and females in video-recorded "mock" job interviews. The professional actors were "normal" weight in one interview. In the second, prostheses made them appear overweight. This experiment also revealed greater hiring bias against overweight women than against overweight men.

Not only is weight included under lookism, but body art modifications such as tattoos and piercings are also included. French et al. (2019), however, found no relationship between tattoos and employability, hiring, wage/salary growth, or any other variable. Cohen et al. (2018), through Emergency Room surveys, found that users of the emergency department services were not concerned if their physicians had tattoos or other body art. (The patients were not informed of the surveys' true purpose.) The surveys indicated that body modifications on an ER physician did not affect the patient's attitude or feelings toward the medical professional. These research findings may represent a shift in beliefs, attitudes, and behaviors in the overall employment market. However, in a pilot study, Drazewski (2013) found that labor market decisionmakers were less likely to hire people with tattoos. Other research related to lookism also demonstrates that many factors can work with sex and race/ethnicity to create healthcare and other workplaces that cannot achieve maximum productivity because of beliefs, attitudes, and behaviors.

In America, "lookism" is not illegal. Some U.S. citizens feel that having body art or colored hair is a form of expression that is protected under the First Amendment as part of the right of freedom of expression. However, private businesses do have the right to implement dress codes that may include no tattoos, piercings, and/or other body art. In early July 2019, California became the first state to ban discrimination against "natural" hairstyles, religious headdresses and other forms of expression when the State passed Senate Bill No. 188 (California Legislative Information, 2019). This Act may be indicative of future changes regarding the operation of lookism as a form of workplace discrimination.

Other Workplace "Isms"

A number of other "Isms" also interact with race/ethnicity and sex. For example, **linguicism** is another factor that operates in workplaces. A linguist, Tove Skutnabb-Kangas (2000), is credited with introducing the concept of linguicism. Linguicism references patterns of beliefs, attitudes, and behaviors that devalue others and reduce their professional and/or personal opportunities because of language. Roth (2019) describes the ability to use the dominant language in a given environment as linguistic capital. The dominant language in U.S. workplaces is not merely English but also English language skills that are compliant with dominant usage patterns. But, language differences can expand into output-inhibiting rather than output-maximizing behaviors. Linguicism can also interact with gender, race/ethnicity, ageism, lookism, and other Isms that affect productivity in healthcare and other workplaces.

Sectarianism is another set of beliefs that may be related to sex and race/ethnicity in healthcare workplaces. In the 1950s, Peter L. Berger (1954) expanded the term "sectarianism" from a definition that references fragmentation within the same religion, to include all fractured groups with their own strongly held beliefs, attitudes, and behaviors. Berger, therefore, widened the definition to apply to other areas of life. Thus, sectarianism does not merely refer to group differences. It describes any situation in which existent values are so important that those with different viewpoints are adversely "judged." While sectarianism is often assigned to the conflicts that occur among groups in other countries, issues such as politics, social stratification, and/or even sports can generate productivity-inhibiting fragmentation in healthcare and other workplaces. Again, sectarianism interacts with the sex and racial/ethnic differences that were listed in Table 1.1. This interaction can cause extreme tension. This tension can then impact diverse workplaces.

Ableism may also impact healthcare and other workplaces. Cherney (2011) highlights the fact that people with disabilities may experience adverse attitudes, beliefs, and behaviors that result in feelings of inferiority and/or superiority. He introduces the term "ableism" to describe this phenomenon. During the past two decades, however, researchers have suggested that by not providing proper accommodations for people with disabilities, society-at-large has contributed to "ableism" (Fougeyrollas et al., 2001; Oliver, 1990). Moreover, Goering (2015) promotes the idea that healthcare professionals should improve their medical practices by gaining further knowledge of the social model of disability as it relates to their patients' needs. Thus, the concept of ableism is another intersectorality that can magnify the impact of sex and/or racial/ethnic bias in healthcare and/or other workplaces.

Nameism (namism) is another intersectionality that may be active in healthcare and non-healthcare workplaces. *Names: A Journal of Onomastics*, which was established in 1952, provides articles on the study of names (American Name Society, n.d.). Marušić (2016) implicitly describes the power of names in a discussion of the problems encountered by scholars with Arabic, Eastern Mediterranean, Chinese, Spanish, and other names. They discovered that such scholars are not properly recognized by journals that utilize American Psychological Association (APA) style and/or other styles that use initials for the first name. Such practices, while intended to be racially/ethnically neutral, can actually transform into nameism in academic healthcare workplaces by suggesting equality gaps in a person's productivity.

Names also denote gender. Therefore, managers and human resource managers who may hold biases against females can activate such biases based upon the use of female-associated names. Hedegaard and Tyran (2018) studied adverse ethnic beliefs, attitudes, and behaviors in workplaces in Denmark. In the experiment, 40 males and 40 females were assigned names that were common in Denmark. In contrast, 46 females and 36 males were assigned Muslim names. The experiment was structured in such a way that participants with non-Danish names were more productive. The results of this experiment revealed that all participants preferred to work with people of their own ethnic background even if such workers were less productive. Thus, it is not surprising that some workers consider changing their names in order to successfully obtain a job. Dr. Mavis Himes (2016) discusses prejudice regarding surnames and first names that "fit" racial or ethnic categories. The article explains why some people feel that employment is more important than keeping their name. In a Swedish study on callbacks made to persons for Assistant Nurse positions, Bursell (2007) found that 60.3% of all applicants were never called back. However, 29.3% of those with Swedish-sounding surnames were recontacted but only 2.6% of persons with other foreign-sounding surnames were called back. Thus, nameism impeded output maximization by dismissing people with certain names from the total employment pool.

▶ How Isms in Healthcare and Other Workplaces Affect Productivity

Table 1.1 is a simple tool with valuable information on the sex/gender and racial/ethnic diversity in healthcare workplaces versus the overall U.S. workplace. However, the workplace is often complicated because each employee has several diverse traits that may affect the person's chances of being hired and/or the worker's experiences with colleagues, managers, and administrators after hiring. These diverse human traits interact when paired with the physical components of a workplace to determine productivity.

Thus, intersectionalities cannot be ignored by a healthcare manager and/or administrator (nor by management in other workplaces). Accordingly, the theme of this handbook is "Isms" in healthcare workplaces. The specific focus is the impact of interactive systems of "Isms" on the healthcare administrator's use of available resources to maximize the services while minimizing the associated costs. In addition to the "Isms" already identified, more common "Isms" may also operate in healthcare and other workplaces such as adverse beliefs, attitudes, and behaviors based on sex, race, religion, sexual preference, and other characteristics. Those Isms negatively impact maximization of output and minimization of costs in healthcare and other workplaces. But, healthcare managers and human resource managers must maximize outcomes and minimize costs and Isms interfere with this mandate.

Before continuing the discussion of Isms in healthcare workplaces, one must ask, "What are these things we call Isms that have been discussed and will continue to be analyzed and described in subsequent chapters of this handbook"?

Definitions of Isms

In some respects, it can be argued that in American society, the single most important source of all word definitions are those reference tools that we call dictionaries. Chen (2012) conducted research on the importance of dictionary use for students learning English as a Second Language (ESL). Hamilton (2012) discusses the importance of dictionary use in learning new vocabulary words in general. Sánchez Ramos (2005) applies practical methods to confirm the power of dictionary use in training people who are learning to become translators. Collier et al. (2016) argue that understanding science, technology, engineering, and mathematics can be improved by applying teaching strategies associated with learning a second language. Thus, there is a rationale for reviewing definitions of Isms and/or other terms from an assortment of dictionaries. **BOX. 1.3** seeks to clarify the term "Isms" by using various dictionaries as a reference point. As Box 1.3 indicates, there are many definitions for "Ism." However, for the purpose of analyzing the **Isms** that are operative in workplaces, we refer to adverse beliefs, attitudes, and behaviors that are directed towards others who are different.

The main focus of healthcare administrators and managers is to plan, direct, organize, monitor, and oversee 20+ million humans in healthcare workplaces and to combine these human resources with available materials, technologies, and financial resources so that outcome maximization can be achieved. The achievement of this task has been made more complex by the different characteristics of workers

---

BOX 1.3 Definitions of "Ism" in Dictionaries

- Ism—a distinctive doctrine, cause, or theory.
  (Courtesy of Merriam-Webster Dictionary. ism. https://www.merriam-webster.com/dictionary/ism Retrieved June 20, 2019.)
- Ism—a set of beliefs, especially ones that one disapproves of.
  (Definition of 'Ism' from Cambridge Dictionary, www.dictionary.cambridge.org, © Cambridge University Press. Used with permission.)

in health care. Healthcare administrators and managers must proactively manage human differences, including those beliefs, attitudes, and behaviors based on these human differences that emerge in diverse healthcare environments. While human differences characterize workplaces worldwide and associated beliefs are attached to these differences, U.S. workplaces also have an extensive assortment of beliefs as a result of the wide range of intersectionalities.

As previously discussed, individuals in workplaces belong to multiple race/ethnicity subgroups. For example, Portuguese Americans are a major subgroup in Bristol County, Massachusetts, and in other areas (U.S. Bureau of Census, 2010). French Canadians are a major subgroup that may be found in the workplaces in Androscoggin County in Maine (U.S. Bureau of Census, 2010). Polish people are a major subgroup in Luzerne County, Pennsylvania, and may be found through-out the businesses in this county (U.S. Bureau of Census, 2004). When the ethnic diversity in the workplace is extended to the country, the mix of backgrounds includes: German Americans (12.6%), Irish Americans (9.4%), Scottish Americans (1.6%), Polish Americans (2.7%), Norwegian Americans (1.3%), Greek Americans (0.4%), Italian Americans (5.0%), Dutch Americans (1.1%), Non–Basque French Americans (2.2%), Swedish Americans (1.1%), Scotch-Irish Americans (.09%), Russian Americans (0.8%), Non-Hispanic West Indian Americans (0.9%), Arab Americans (.6%), and others (U.S. Census Bureau, 2018). Additionally, workplaces in the United States include Non-Hispanic African Americans (12.7%), Mexican Americans of all races (11.3%), Cuban (0.7%), Puerto Rican Americans of any race 1.8%, Chinese Americans (1.3%), Asian Indian Americans (1.3%), and numerous other groups (American Community Survey, 2018).

Similarly, there are 562 federally recognized Native American tribes including 229 Alaskan native tribes who are actively employed in one workplace or another. Asian Americans in U.S. workplaces include Chinese, Filipinos, Indians, Vietnamese, Korean, Japanese, Taiwanese, or other Asian (for example, Pakistani, Cambodians, Hmong, Thai, Laotians, Bangladeshi, Burmese, Indonesians, Sri Lankans, Malaysians, Bhutanese, Mongolians, Okinawans, etc.) Africans and other immigrants who speak Igbo, Arabic, Hausa, Spanish, Akon, Yoruba, French, Wolof, or other languages, also work in U.S. healthcare and other workplaces. While the Census Bureau had stopped collecting data on ethnic diversity, the ancestry question were once again included in the 2020 census (U.S. Bureau of Census, 2020). A decision in a 1987 court case, Saint Francis College vs. Al-Khazraji, was considered a precursor for the return of the question (Oyez, 2018).

Healthcare environments, like other U.S. workplaces, are also religiously diverse. More than 310 different religions are represented (Whalen, 1981). The spectrum includes atheists, agnostics, neopaganists, and others. Christianity, Islam, Hinduism, Buddhism, Sikhism, Judaism, and other religions are represented.

U.S. workplaces and healthcare workplaces are also diverse along other variables. These include workers with different types of "intelligences," various "gender identities," and other factors. Accordingly, this handbook briefly examines healthcare workplaces and identifies how to increase productivity and positive outcomes. The purpose of this treastise is that of reducing the presence of workplace Isms in order to promote productivity, resource maximization, and performance goal achievement.

A Portrait of Healthcare Workplaces

Healthcare professionals are asked to maximize productivity in a complex environment. Phillip (2016) describes the healthcare workplace as having a high potential for workplace violence. In other words, while healthcare workplaces focus on the remediation of illness and disease, healthcare employees work in an environment in which the risks of violence may be even higher than commonly believed because the number and magnitude of these incidents is often under-reported. According to Phillip's statistics (2016), healthcare environments rank next to law enforcement in terms of employers' risks of violence-related injury or death. The sources of violence range from verbal assault, sexual assault, to actual death.

The U.S. Department of Labor's publication, Occupational Safety and Health Administration publication, *Workplace Violence in Healthcare: Understanding the Challenge* (2015), argues that physical violence, threats of violence, verbally abusive behavior, multiple forms of harassment, and other threats occur 400% more often in the healthcare industry than in the retail, manufacturing, and other workplaces. A study by Wong et al. (2019) in the Joint Commission's Journal on Quality and Patient Safety also has similar findings.

Not only must healthcare workers be concerned about their own safety, they must also protect the patients. However, Wong et al. found that healthcare workers are at even greater risk than their patients. These authors also argue that workplace violence has not been adequately addressed. In a study of the higher risk of workplace violence against nurses in emergency departments, Li et al. (2019) confirmed that such circumstances decrease output maximization by increasing job dissatisfaction and the potential for job turnover.

Workplace violence and threats of violence are directed toward healthcare workers from a multitude of sources, i.e., patients, friends, and/or family members of patients and visitors. Unfortunately, coworkers also threaten and/or actually assault other coworkers. Such circumstances create additional duties for healthcare administrators that range far beyond the realm of financial, logistical, managerial, and other traditional "business" duties. Healthcare administrators and managers are expected to gather analytics on the prevalence and nature of such incidents. However, the healthcare administrator must also assess subpopulation health issues associated with these incidents. Finally, the healthcare administrator must ensure that healthcare workers are properly diagnosed regarding their injuries and that they receive the best possible treatment after experiencing actual and/or threats of violence.

Workplace violence against healthcare workers is not new nor does it occur only in U.S. healthcare work environments. Gates (2004) labeled this phenomenon as an "epidemic" more than a decade ago. Brophy et al. (2018) introduced the claim that in Canadian healthcare workplaces, violence against healthcare workers has now become commonplace. Mann (2018) also found that nurses are particularly at risk. But Joshi and Joshi (2018) informs us that in India, junior physicians feel that they are at a higher risk of violence than is the case with their senior-level colleagues. Based on small group discussions, physicians believe that the absence of protection, patient distance, and a greater shift toward nonhumanitarian values may be partially responsible for the growing violence.

Bar-David (2018), in an inquiry into workplace violence in Israel, does not examine violence in healthcare workplaces as an independent phenomenon. Rather, this author emphasizes that a workplace which permits workers to engage in behaviors that can be categorized as "workplace incivilities," has allowed more aggressive violence to be introduced. Stated differently, **workplace Isms**, a primary cause of "workplace incivilities," may be at fault.

The impact of this violence is decreased output. Gerberich et al. (2004) conducted a survey on the impact of physical violence and incivility in the workplace. By using a sample of 6,300 RNs and LPNs, they found that the consequences of incivilities are as great as when physical assaults occur. It must be reiterated that workplace violence impedes the work of healthcare administrators and managers by generating employee turnover.

Choi and Lee (2017) confirmed that nurses in Korea who experienced workplace violence often decided to leave their jobs. Call et al. (2014) found that in the retail industry, turnover rate changes can lead to "changes in performance." Konings and Vanormelingen (2015) also demonstrated that turnover can diminish productivity even more when on-the-job and/or external training has occurred among those workers who leave a worksite.

Some evidence exists that in healthcare workplaces, as in other industries, diversity itself is associated with problems. Mikkonen et al. (2016) found that even culturally and linguistically diverse students who work in healthcare workplaces are often underestimated in terms of their capabilities. Van Ryn et al. (2015) reported that medical students of varied races/ethnicities sometimes develop implicit racial bias based on having heard negative comments from attending physicians about African American patients. Based on an analysis of personal narratives, Sue et al. (2007) discovered that healthcare work environments frequently include unconscious "micro-aggressions" among Caucasian supervisors, managers, etc., and other workers.

Sue et al.'s research revealed that three forms of **micro-aggression** may operate within healthcare and other environments. **Micro-assault** references actions that are overt phenomena of subgroup discrimination. It may involve the use of harsh words and language or other intentional acts. **Micro-insults** involve negative statements regarding an individual's subgroup. **Micro-invalidation** involves behaviors and/or statements that dismiss the thoughts, feelings, and/or beliefs of an individual from another subgroup. Sue et al.'s research revealed continual instances of one or more of the above behaviors in the counseling-based healthcare environment in which the study was conducted. While the original study applies these terms to acts involving racial/ethnic diversity, we apply the concepts to all subgroups whether based on religion, sexual minority status, gender, country of origin, language group, rural/urban status, age, and/or any other subgroup of workers who are bullied and/or demeaned in workplaces characterized by heterogeneity rather than homogeneity. The demeaning of the individual can be based on attractiveness (lookism), age (ageism), and/or a range of other Isms. Even individuals considered "nerds" comprise an identifiable subgroup.

Whitgob et al. (2016) discuss another problem that healthcare administrators and managers may need to address. This problem is discrimination against a diverse physician by a patient and his family. These researchers also provide tips on how Stanford University medical students were equipped to address such problems in the workplace through a process of intense training. Reynolds et al. (2015) outline appropriate workplace behaviors for both physicians and administrators when patients reject services from diverse physicians. In contrast, Paul-Emile et al. (2016) explore the complicated legal and ethical issues in healthcare workplaces when patients reject services delivered by a diverse physician or other healthcare professional. For example, legal cases have been brought against medical institutions that "removed" a healthcare worker from attending to a patient based on the patient's specific request to not be treated by a medical professional of a certain race or ethnicity. Thus, research on healthcare workplaces demonstrates that multiple Isms exist and must be addressed by healthcare managers and administrators.

For example, studies have revealed that when the diversity in the healthcare environment is based on sex, patients prefer males. Freedman (2010) introduces evidence to support this finding. **Nameism** as discussed earlier, was operative in a research study conducted by Greene, Hibbard, and Sacks (2018). These researchers, in a study of 915 patients, found that the name of a physician can lead to implicit bias. Specifically, this study revealed that the name of a physician who was seemingly a White American male was more frequently selected by the participants than the names that suggested an African American male, an African American female, a White American woman, or a Middle Eastern physician of unknown gender. Huraib et al. (2015) uncovered data that revealed that women in Riyadh who were surveyed regarding dentist selection favored male dentists. Cydulka et al. (2000) cite findings regarding a preference for males in emergency medical environments. Heaton and Marquez (1990) surveyed males regarding physician preferences for male genitalia exams. Over one-half of the study group indicated a preference for a male provider for the genital portion of the exam and 61.5% preferred the same for the rectal portion of the exam. Yet, zero participants indicated a preference for a female provider for either of these exams. This suggests that there may be a relationship between type of treatment and sexual preference for a male physician.

Other studies have found that medical specialty areas can also influence physician gender preferences by patients. For example, Chandler, Chandler, and Dabbs (2000) found that female patients preferred a female Ob/Gyn because they felt that female doctors could better understand their medical issues. Tobler et al. (2016) performed research that produced similar results. In an analysis of gender preference studies, these researchers uncovered the fact that over one-half of the patients preferred a female Ob/Gyn. Also, a study conducted by Shamrani (2016) revealed that over 250 women reported partiality toward a female medical professional in the area of Ob/Gyn care, gynecological surgery, and infant care. These same women also preferred a female physician for their general health appointments.

Interestingly, in a study conducted by Van Ness and Lynch (2000), male youth also preferred female physicians when it involved general physical examinations. Approximately half of the youth also indicated a preference for a female physician to perform a genital examination. Moreover, researchers Kim, Kang, and Kwon (2017) found that female patients had a preference for same-sex urologists. Other results revealed that approximately 65% of male participants in the study who had a preference preferred a male urologist. A *JAMA* article also states that just under 100% of females who responded to a survey preferred female dermatologists to test for skin cancer whereas only 37.5% of the males did so (Houston, et al., 2016).

Similar trends have been noted for over three decades. For example, researchers Fennema, Meyer, and Owen (1990) conducted a survey among a small sample of adult patients regarding family medical services. The results revealed that just under half indicated that they preferred one gender over another. For those who did so, over 40% of the female respondents and 12% of the males indicated a preference for a female physician and 31% of the men who had a gender preference were inclined to prefer a male physician.

Patients' preferences for a physician of a specific gender have also been cited as a barrier to health-related processes. For example, Menees and Inadomi (2005) surveyed 202 adult women and found that 43% of them preferred a same-sex endoscopist for a colon check. However, many of the women were willing to postpone this important wellness check for 30 or more days to ensure that they could see a female physician. This can directly result in the delay of the discovery of any abnormalities and, as a result, place the patient's health at risk. As can be seen, physician gender preference is a well-researched area but one whose results are also varied. The data collected from these types of surveys can inform the health community of specific attitudes concerning certain procedures and screenings. This information can then be used to decrease patient decisions that could delay important health screenings and/or care. In such cases, the public health sector can provide support by reducing genderism before it becomes a problem in healthcare workplaces. It can be said that patients in healthcare workplaces mimics the mechanisms of the American workplace in general.

In the past, healthcare workplaces have relied on cultural diversity training to improve problems associated with diversity. Anand and Winters (2008) identified three primary phases in developing cultural diversity training over the three decades before the publication of their research.

Phase 1 was defined as the mid-1960s to the early 1980s. The Civil Rights Act of 1964 (Pub. L. 88-352, 78 stat. 241) was passed during this period (Pedriana and Stryker, 2004). While this broad-based law focused on several areas, workplace discrimination was included under its auspices. Whether the basis of exclusion was race/ethnicity, sex, religion, country of origin, and/or other, such subgroup stratifiers could no longer be applied to these social institutions nor to any programs that received financial assistance from the federal government. Title VII of the Civil Rights Act of 1964 established the Equal Employment Opportunity Commission (EEOC) to oversee the enforcement of this Act.

While the passage of this law affected all workplaces with more than 15 workers, healthcare work environments were particularly impacted. Friedman (2014) cites data on the hospital workplaces that existed *prior to* the Civil Rights Act of 1964. **BOX 1.4** lists some practices carried out by hospital administrators and managers.

After the passage of the Civil Rights Act of 1964, workers were given cultural diversity training to promote compliance with the new legislation prohibiting workplace discrimination. Stated differently, the training was primarily designed to enhance compliance with the newly passed legislation. However, as a result of such training, the unique race-based Isms that existed in hospitals via patients and hospital staff decreased dramatically.

BOX 1.4   An Overview of Hospitals as Employment and Health Delivery Sites Before the Civil Rights Act of 1964

- Approximately 83% of hospitals in northern states accepted all races/ethnicities but only 6% of hospitals in southern states did so.
- Approximately ⅓ of the 94% of the nonintegrated hospitals in the South were workplaces that provided no health care to African Americans and limited care to people of other ethnicities.
- Approximately ½ of the nonintegrated southern hospitals did serve African American patients but did so in separate, nonintegrated areas of the hospitals.
- Relative to employment, approximately 90% of northern hospitals did not provide training to African American interns and researchers.
- Approximately 94% of southern hospitals also similarly excluded African American employees.
- Interestingly, approximately 80% of northern hospitals granted staff privileges to non-Caucasian physicians, but a mere 5% of southern hospitals granted staff privileges to non-Caucasian physicians.

Modified from Friedman, E. (2014). U.S. Hospital and the Civil Rights Act of 1964. Hospitals of Health Networks; Smith, D. B. (1988). The racial segregation of hospital care revisited, *American Journal of Public Health, 88*(3), 461–463.

In addition, adverse beliefs, attitudes, and behaviors also impact other races/ethnicities. A considerable body of research indicates that both in the past and present, Asian American students have had difficulty being accepted to undergraduate, graduate, and professional school programs at highly selective colleges/universities due to external, internal, and institutionalized biases (Asian-American Coalition for Education, 2018). Despite such circumstances, Asian Americans now comprise 19.8% of all physicians and surgeons in the country (U.S. Department of Labor, Bureau of Labor Statistics, 2018). Similarly, despite negative reactions to people of Islamic faith, although Muslims are only 1% of the American population, they are over-represented among physicians and surgeons. However, some patients in healthcare workplaces still refuse services by diverse physicians. Moreover, both Asian American and Muslim American physicians believe that healthcare workplaces may still demonstrate a lack of ethnic balance in their workplace practices. Such findings are also reflected in the popular literature. Science News (2015) published an article on discrimination against Muslim-American physicians.

In a Washington Post article, Kristine Phillips (August 21, 2017) reported on a patient's refusal to receive care from an award-winning, emergency room physician in Portland, Oregon because of race/ethnicity and sex. Similarly, Jacqueline Howard (October 26, 2016) reported on the experience of a young intern at Lucile Packard Children's Hospital at Stanford University. The article reports that the father of this young patient examined the intern's nametag. The father's response was, according to the author, "Oh, is that a Jewish last name? I don't want a Jewish doctor." In 2017, a video of a frustrated woman in line at an emergency clinic asking that her son be treated by a physician of a particular race went viral. Many other examples could be cited.

Phase 2 in the effort to address workplace Isms was quite different from the mechanisms that prevailed during Phase 1. Phase 2 was defined by Anand and Winters (2008) as the mid-1980s to the mid-1990s. This phase was less directed toward the new law and workplace education regarding the consequences of its implementation. Rather, the emphasis was on improving the ability of diverse employees to work together. Thus, the focus was on diversity in workplaces. The reason for the shift to Phase 2 workplace interventions was simple. During this period, cultural differences created workplace misunderstandings. Workplaces are, of course, always affected by the overall economy. During the mid-1980s, the U.S. labor market in general had a number of characteristics which increased competition for jobs. Toossi (2002) describes some of these changes listed in **BOX 1.5**.

BOX 1.5 The American Labor Market : 1980s to 1990s

- From 1950 to 1960, civilian labor force participation rates grew from 59.2% of all people age 16 and older to 59.4%—an increase of less than 1% (.67%).
- From 1970 to 1980, labor force participation rates increased from 60.4% to 63.8%—a growth rate of 5.62%.
- From 1980 to 1990, this trend continued and the labor force participation rate increased to 66.4%—an additional increase of 4.07%. Thus, there was greater competition for jobs.
- Overall, the composition of the labor force changed:
  - Women, a group who had an overall civilian labor force participation rate of 33.9% in 1950, had a labor force participation rate of 51.5% by 1980 and 57.5% by 1990.
  - Thus, by 1980, this group had added gender diversity to the workplace via a 51.9% growth in their labor force participation rates and by an additional growth rate of 11.15% by 1990. Racial/ethnic diversity had also increased. While the Department of Labor did not track civilian labor force participation rates for these groups until 1980, labor force participation rates were 64.6% for Asian Americans in 1980, 61.0% for African Americans, and 64.0% for Hispanic/Latino Americans.
  - By 1990, the labor force participation rates of African Americans (63.3%), Asian Americans (65.4%), and Latinos (67%) had grown even more. Accordingly, racial/ethnic diversity in the workplace had increased.
- In addition, an era of industry shifts had occurred (Plunkert, 1990).
  - Mining employment had dropped by 25%.
  - Manufacturing employment had decreased by 7%.
  - Construction employment had increased by 19%.
  - Government, transportation, and public utilities had experienced an 11% increase in employment.
- However, health care, business, and general services experienced explosive growth.
  - Retail trade had a 30% increase in employment.
  - Finance, insurance, and real estate's employment had increased by 37%.
  - Health services employment grew by 52.9% and social services, an allied field, increased its employment by 49.5%. Such changes brought greater numbers of women and minorities into a service economy that included greater customer/employee contact.

Modified from Toossi, M. (2002). A century of change: The US labor force, 1950–2050. *Monthly Lab. Rev., 125*, 15.

Additionally, with increased labor force participation rates and the changing structure of the labor force, it is less than surprising that **structural unemployment** occurred, thereby increasing overall unemployment rates.

TABLE 1.2 compares unemployment rates from 1980 to 1995 with the rates that existed in 1970.

TABLE 1.2 Unemployment Rates in 1980–1995 (Reference 1970)		
Year	**%**	**% Change Relative to 1970**
1970	4.9	Baseline
1980	7.1	+44.89
1981	7.6	+55.10
1982	9.7	+97.95
1983	9.6	+95.91
1984	7.5	+53.06
1985	7.2	+46.93
1986	7.0	+42.85
1987	6.2	+26.53
1988	5.5	+12.24
1989	5.3	+8.16
1990	5.6	+14.28
1991	6.8	+38.77
1992	7.5	+53.06
1993	6.9	+40.81
1994	6.1	+24.48
1995	5.6	+14.28

Data from United States Department of Labor, Bureau of Labor Statistics, Database Tables & Calculations, Labor Force Statistics from the current population survey, series I.D.: LNU04000000. Unemployment Rate, Percent or rate 16 years and over 1947–2017, Data extracted on August 1, 2019. https://data.bls.gov/timeseries/LNU04000000?periods=Annual+Data&periods_option=specific _periods&years_option=all_years

As Table 1.2 indicates, the early and mid-1980s and the early-1990s were characterized by significant increases in unemployment relative to 1970. Simultaneously, when these economic conditions were accompanied by public policies such as affirmative action, increased data collection on employment statistics, and other related matters, increasing conflict occurred regarding the value added by diverse labor markets. Yet, Herring (2009), using data from 1996 and 1997 from the National Organizations Survey, tested several workplace hypotheses and found that racial/ethnic diversity was positively related to an enlarged customer base, higher sales revenue, growth in market share, and increased profits. Similarly, gender diversity in the workplace was also associated with an augmented customer base, higher overall revenues, and profit augmentation.

However, workers were not aware of such findings. Accordingly, by the mid-80s and into the mid-90s, the emphasis on diversity was associated with conflict in the various workplaces. In fact, workers were absolutely unaware that diversity made such an impact. Yet, Wright et al.'s (2017) analysis of data from 1986 to 1992 found that successful affirmative action programs, when announced by the U.S. Department of Labor for awards, had the power to increase the value of a company's stock. This was because the potential losses associated with discrimination-related lawsuit settlements reduced the value of a company's stock. While managers and administrators *were aware* of such outcomes, it is not surprising that these managers began using cultural diversity training during this period with a focus on a reduction in diversity-related workplace conflict.

Numerous diversity-related settlements have been and continue to be awarded in health care. As recently as June 25, 2019, a Michigan-based healthcare company was ordered to pay $74,418 in response to a religious discrimination lawsuit (EEOC Press Release, 2019). On February 28, 2018 (Rege, 2018), it was reported that a general damages award was made for $630,000 and a $3.2 million punitive damages award was made against a hospital in Hawaii because hospital administrators and managers couldn't eliminate harassment and negative treatment by coworkers. Gehring (2017) reported a discrimination case regarding a child who committed suicide after experiencing imperfect services at Rady Children's Hospital because of bias against transgenders. More cases of this type will occur because Title VI of the Civil Rights Act of 1964 has been specifically extended to the area of health care and human services. Section 504 of the Rehabilitation Act of 1973 (Rehab Act), Title II of the American Disabilities Act (ADA), Section 1557 of the Patient Protection and Affordable Care Act (ACA or ObamaCare), and the Genetic Information Non-Discrimination Act of 2008 (GINA) also apply to healthcare workplaces. Matthew (2015) provides an excellent overview of healthcare cases of discrimination over recent and past history. However, a review of cases on healthcare law and diversity reveals the greater complexity of filing and winning cases in this area. This factor further justifies cultural diversity training in seeking to decrease diversity-related workplace conflict.

Phase 3, which is the 21st century, has now arrived. Phase 3 differs from the past experiences with workplace Isms in that there is now greater proactivity. Specifically, overall efforts now seek to advance strategies that will make the "whole stronger than the sum of its parts." Thus, Phase 3 focuses on ensuring that America's culturally diverse workplaces benefit the country and the world. This has not been the historical approach. Thus, before looking at America's culturally diverse workforce of today and tomorrow, it is helpful to examine the past.

The History of Isms in American Labor Markets

Isms in American workplaces are integrated throughout American history. Irish Americans are a great example. Irish Americans' integration into the American workplace had many problems because of ethnic and religious diversity. For example, in 1831, Protestants burned down St. Mary's Catholic Church to protest Catholics' presence in America and in the workplace (Hoeber, 2001). In 1844, approximately 13 Irish immigrants died in a riot that Americans of other ethnicities initiated in order to protect their workplaces from hiring Irish Americans. In 1854, policies to include the Irish into the society and the workplace were shut down by the American Party's refusal to allow the Irish to participate in party activities. Alzughaibi (2015) uses historical literature to understand the cultural diversity that penetrated the American workplace and American life. Indeed, although some scholars deny it, "NO IRISH NEED APPLY" signs were on the windows and facades of many American workplaces (Lind, 2015). As a result, members of this culturally diverse group were excluded from higher-paying jobs in the workplace and, in some cases, experienced demotions.

However, Irish Americans were not the only immigrant group subjected to such injustices. Chinese immigrants who came to America in the mid-1860s to help build railroads also endured racial intolerance and discrimination. Many were beaten, killed, robbed, and tortured because they were different from their attackers (Library of Congress, 2019). In 1875, the United States passed the Page Act (1875). This legislation stopped Chinese women from immigrating to the country because they were the subjects of cheap labor and were labeled immoral (Peffer, 1986). This Act was soon followed by the passage of the Chinese Exclusion Act (1882), which stated that no new Chinese immigrants were allowed into the country for the next decade. This Act became a permanent law in 1902. It was not repealed until 1943 (Teaching for Diversity and Social Justice, 2007).

Mexican Americans were also subjected to ethnic discrimination after the United States won the Mexican American war and entered into the Treaty of Guadalupe Hidalgo (1848). The United States purchased the land from Mexico. This land now comprises the states of California, Texas, Utah, New Mexico, Arizona, and Nevada. The United States allowed the citizens of Mexico's territory to become U.S. citizens. They were also allowed to keep their land but discovered that providing proof of ownership was difficult for many reasons (Zinn, 1990). Language barriers, the requirement that all ownership matters be managed by an American-appointed commission, lack of accurate border designations, and other challenges occurred. Some claimants were even required to surrender up to 25% of their land in exchange for services to American lawyers. Moreover, other claimants took out high-interest loans in their attempts to provide ownership. These types of circumstances resulted in a large number of landowners losing their land. The Treaty also eventually resulted in the Mexican and American residents of the new American territory being segregated.

Higher education is, of course, linked to workplace success. Fordham University (Schroth, 2008) and Boston College emerged as educational institutions to educate Irish Americans and thus advance their inclusion in U.S. labor markets (Boston College, 2018). Numerous other culturally diverse groups have also experienced barriers to workforce inclusion throughout American history.

Molnar (2010) describes problems of workplace diversity that excluded Italian immigrants from many workplaces because of the perception that they were not physically strong. However, this discrimination even extended to Italian immigrants whose educational levels qualified them for placement in higher-level positions involving nonphysical work. In an article by Henegham (2012), a quote is included by President Harry S. Truman as part of a plea for greater workforce inclusion. President Truman stated:

> *"The idea behind this discriminatory policy was, to put it boldly, that Americans with English or Irish names were better people and better citizens than Americans with Italian or Greek or Polish names. It was thought that people of Western Europe made better citizens than Rumanians or Yugoslavs or Ukrainians or Hungarians or Balts or Austrians. Such a concept is utterly unworthy of our traditions and our ideals. It violates the great political doctrine of the Declaration of Independence that "all men are created equal." (pg. 1787)*

Again, such responses to human differences also occur globally. Daldy et al. (2013) report on diversity issues in New Zealand workplaces. They describe Asian and Pacific-Islander immigrants of higher education in New Zealand as the group who most often experience adverse workplace beliefs, attitudes, and behaviors. Similarly, Siklossy (2018) describes a gloomy picture of diversity problems in Europe. **BOX 1.6** lists some of the issues identified.

Given the apparent universality of such behaviors, workplaces in American society cannot legally exclude culturally diverse groups. These generalized adverse behaviors based on human differences also explain why laws, policies, community-based efforts, and individuals often oppose acts that do not contribute to the advancement of humankind.

BOX 1.6 Problems of Cultural Diversity in European Workplaces

- Applicants for jobs in Belgium are nearly ⅓ less likely to be invited for job interviews if their names suggest that they are not Belgian.
- Explicit government laws, regulations, and policies support disparate outcomes in some workplaces.
- Asymmetric employee recruitment mechanisms and processes generate higher levels of unemployment for religious and ethnic minorities.
- Diverse employees earn less, have shorter job tenures, and experience more workplace instances of explicit and/or implicit bias, etc.
- In Ireland, approximately 31% of all racial/ethnic acts occur within workplaces.
- Italy and Greece practice extreme disregard for the humanity of migrant workers.
- In France, Cyprus, Belgium, and other countries, women in the workplace are at high risk of violence, sexual harassment, and sexual abuse.

Modified from European Network Against Racism (2018). Press Release: No progress in curbing racial discrimination in the European labour market – in particular for women of colour. https://www.enar-eu.org/No-progress-in-curbing-racial-discrimination-in-the-European-labour-market-in-1490

Human Differences in Healthcare Workplaces

While data on employment and health and social services have already been presented, it becomes important to more closely examine patterns that may be directed toward diverse groups in American healthcare markets. As **TABLE 1.3** reveals, the physician marketplace is changing.

Table 1.3 reveals a trend of an increased representation of females within hospitals, group practices, private practices, and other physician workplaces. Specifically, females were 33.5% of all active physicians in 2016. That number has increased annually since that time. **TABLE 1.4** provides data on sex and race/ethnicity in healthcare occupations for 2018.

As Table 1.4 reveals, healthcare labor markets are considerably more diverse than is generally known. For example, while females are 46.9% of the overall workforce, they are 72.0% of the administrators and managers in healthcare workplaces. Thus, females are over-represented by 53.51%. In addition, the proportion of Americans of European descent is represented among healthcare administrators and managers by a percent that is less than their representation in the overall workforce. African Americans are 11.5% of medical service administrators and managers. This group is 12.3% of the overall workforce. In contrast, Asian Americans are under-represented among medical and health service managers by 26%. Finally, Latinx Americans are under-represented among healthcare administrators and managers by 52.02%. Overall, such data reveal that healthcare workplaces are extremely diverse.

However, healthcare workers are unevenly distributed not only by the type of healthcare workplaces described in Table 1.1 but also by the type of positions held in these workplaces. Table 1.4 specifically lists the total number of people who work as healthcare providers. It also highlights the percent distribution of these providers in healthcare workplaces by gender and race/ethnicity. (No current data have yet been compiled that categorize healthcare practitioners by the full range of stratifiers such as age, religion, physical limitations, sexual preferences, and other categories that have developed into workplace Isms.) **BOX 1.7** provides interpretations of some of the data in Table 1.4.

It is important to note that under-representation and/or over-representation alone does not necessarily mean that Isms exist at work. Such conclusions can represent different occupational preference functions relative to work, intergenerational occupational patterns, and/or other variables. In a classic article, Brewster and Rindfuss (2000) advance the long-standing conclusion that preferences regarding fertility and child-bearing may have an influence on the occupational choices of women. Bitner's (1992) research implies that the physical environment of various healthcare occupations may generate differentiated occupational choices and a varied emphasis on work security can impact occupational choice (Heejung and Mau, 2014). In contrast, Gallie (2019) describes how occupational choices can reflect different norms and preferences at work. However, one measure that indicates the impact of Isms is different pay for the same work. Accordingly, it becomes important to examine whether healthcare workplaces are characterized by inequalities in pay.

TABLE 1.3 A Profile of Physician Diversity in Healthcare Workplaces, 2010–2016

Actively Licensed Physicians	Physicians by Gender					
	2010		2016			
	Count	%	Count	%	% Change	
■ Male	583,315	68.6	617,186	64.7	–5.6	
■ Female	252,861	29.7	319,145	33.5	12.79	
■ Unknown	13,909	1.6	17,364	1.8	12.5	
Total:	**850,085**	**100**	**953,695**	**100**	**11.21**	

Data from Young, A., Chaudhry, H. J., Pei, X., Arnhart, K., Dugan, M., & Snyder, G. B. (2017). A census of actively licensed physicians in the United States, 2016. *Journal of Medical Regulation, 103*(2), 7–21.

TABLE 1.4 Gender and Race/Ethnicity by Occupations: 2018

Occupation	Total Employed	% Women	% White Americans	% African Americans	% Asian Americans	% Hispanic/ Latino Americans
All Industry Occupations	**155,761,000**	**46.9**	**78.0**	**12.3**	**6.3**	**17.3**
Medical Health Services Managers	**639,000**	**72.0**	**80.9**	**11.5**	**5.0**	**9.0**
Healthcare Practitioners and Technical Occupations	**9,420,000**	**75.0**	**75.2**	**12.6**	**9.9**	**8.5**
-Chiropractors	63,000	21.1	92.8	0.9	4.0	3.0
-Dentists	162,000	35.7	79.0	1.6	17.6	4.3
-Dietitians and Nutritionists	104,000	93.1	78.6	9.6	9.1	9.6
-Optometrists	54,000	46.0	84.9	2.1	9.1	8.5
-Pharmacists	348,000	63.4	67.9	7.2	23.1	4.4
-Physicians & Surgeons	1,094,000	40.3	70.8	7.6	19.8	7.4

(continues)

TABLE 1.4 Gender and Race/Ethnicity by Occupations: 2018   *(continued)*

Occupation	Total Employed	% Women	% White Americans	% African Americans	% Asian Americans	% Hispanic/ Latino Americans
-Physician Assistants	132,000	72.1	90.3	2.9	5.1	8.2
-Podiatrists	11,000	-	-	-	-	-
-Audiologists	10,000	-	-	-	-	-
-Occupational Therapists	116,000	86.8	91.1	2.5	6.4	4.2
-Physical Therapy	286,000	69.5	76.4	7.4	14.3	4.3
-Radiation Therapists	16,000	-	-	-	-	-
-Respiratory Therapists	108,000	63.8	64.9	17.3	13.9	11.6
-Registered Nurses	3,213,000	88.6	75.5	13.1	9.0	7.2
-Nurse Practitioners	212,000	87.2	79.1	11.2	8.8	2.6

Data from U.S. Department of Labor, Bureau of Labor Statistics, 2018, Table 11. Employed Persons by detailed occupation, sex, race, and Hispanic or Latino Ethnicity. https://www.bls.gov/cps/cpsaat11.pdf

---

BOX 1.7 Asymmetrical Patterns of Employment Among Healthcare Providers by Sex and Race/Ethnicity

Female Healthcare Workers by Occupation

- Females were 93.1% of dietitians and nutritionists. Thus, women work as Dietitians and Nutritionists at a rate that is 98.5% higher than their representation in the overall workforce.
- Approximately 87.2% of nurse practitioners were female. This exceeds their representation in the health practitioner and technical operator marketplaces by 16.26% and their representation in the overall workplace by 85.93%.
- Women were 40.3% of physicians and surgeons. Thus, they were under-represented among physicians and surgeons by 56.16%, given the fact that they were 75% of all people who are healthcare practitioners and technical operators.

Healthcare Workers by Race/Ethnicity and Sex Combined

- African Americans, a group who were 12.6% of all healthcare practitioners, were under-represented in most healthcare practitioner and technical operator occupations except respiratory therapists (17.3%), registered nurses (13.1%), clinical laboratory technologists and technicians (18.6%), health practitioners, support technologists and technicians (14.1%), and medical records and health information technicians (15.5%). However, this group was also over-represented in the number of licensed practical and licensed vocational nurses (30.4%).
- Asian Americans, a racial/ethnic group who were 9.9% of healthcare practitioners and technical operators, were significantly over-represented as dentists (17.6%), pharmacists (23.1%), physicians and surgeons (19.8%), physical therapists (14.3%), respiratory therapists (13.9%), and miscellaneous health technologists and technicians (14.4%).
- Latinx Americans, a group who were 17.3% of the population, were under-represented in all healthcare provider occupations including dentists (4.3%), pharmacists (4.4%), physicians and surgeons (7.4%), physician assistants (8.2%), registered nurses (7.2%), Nurse Practitioners (2.6%), and other occupations.

Data from U.S. Department of Labor, Bureau of Labor Statistics, 2018, Table 11. Employed Persons by detailed occupation, sex, race, and Hispanic or Latino Ethnicity. https://www.bls.gov/cps/cpsaat11.pdf

Earning Differentials

A number of studies have found that healthcare work environments may be characterized by statistically significant pay differences by gender. Kavilanz (2018) reports recent data from an organization called Doximity. Based on this report, physicians, as a group, not only experience higher overall earnings but also higher wage growth than the overall workforce. Physicians' work efforts led to a 4% increase in income relative to 2.6% for the economy as a whole in 2017. Thus, in that year, physician incomes grew 53.84% faster than the increase for workers as a whole. However, the survey data revealed that female physicians earned, on average, 28% less than male physicians.

Before concluding that Isms are responsible, one must first ask, "Is Doximity a reliable source of such data"? Doximity, unlike the American Medical Association, is a social networking online community of physicians. Approximately 65,000 licensed physicians participated in the survey on which the data are based. Thus, Doximity

---

BOX 1.8 Disparities in Gender Physician Earnings by Geographical Area and Medical Specialty

The 2017 survey data by Doximity revealed that:

- The gender earnings gap for physicians increased from $91,254 in 2016 to $105,000 in 2017—an increase of 15.02% in 1 year.
- Significant differentials existed in every single medical specialty and in every single geographic area included in the survey.
- Relative to medical specialties, women in orthopedic surgery who participated in the survey earned $101,291 less than their male counterparts—the greatest income differential by area and specialty.
- However, women in occupational medicine earned $59,174 less than their male counterparts.
- Charleston, South Carolina, was the geographic marketplace in the survey with the highest gender/sex-based earning differential—$134,499.

Data from Kavilanz, P. (2018). The Gender Pay Gap For Women Doctors Is Big – And Getting Worse. Money.cnn.com, accessed May 14, 2018.

---

is a primary source of primary data and, as a result, is considered a reliable and valid source of physician data. Accordingly, **BOX 1.8** provides greater detail on the Doximity report regarding the earning disparities among physicians in the healthcare marketplace.

Other data also reveal that a number of pay disparities in healthcare workplaces exist. Moore et al. (2016) analyzed data from the 2008 National Sample Survey of Registered Nurses. These analysts identified interesting trends. Asian American nurses earned significantly greater salaries than White American nurses. African American and Latinx American nurses had lower earnings than their White American counterparts. Moreover, these earning gaps were not explainable by differentials in experience or other factors. Specifically, these researchers were unable to identify differences in education, years of experience, or other rational causes of earning discrepancies. However, it is important to note that numerous other forces may be at play ranging from personal factors to different styles of communication to differences in the occupational duties completed by these nurses (Spetz, 2016). Numerous other articles also confirm the type of problems that occur in culturally diverse workplaces. However, the purpose of this text is not to propagate controversy. Rather, the objective of this handbook is to provide input to the question, "How can diversity in healthcare workplaces be addressed by healthcare administrators and managers in order to maximize workplace outcomes"?

▶ Diverse Worker Characteristics and Outcome Maximization

The primary tool used in American workplaces to maximize positive outcomes is employee training. This strategy emerged, in part, because the EEOC has been an advocate for such training. Indeed, both healthcare and other workplaces typically provide online and/or in-class didactic training on what the federal government considers lawful and/or unlawful actions. Additionally, most workplaces include written employee handbooks and manuals that cover federal and state laws regarding expected behaviors in workplaces. These materials inform workers of the employer's overall guidelines and expectations of those who serve as employees or contractors. Not only do these materials promote employee and employer compliance with Title VII and Title VI of the federal law, they also address diversity protection laws at the state and local levels. Oftentimes, administrators and managers in workplaces complement the distribution of written materials with mandatory online training. These steps are taken because workplaces today are more diverse than ever.

As discussed, such differences may be based on language, race/ethnicity, nationality, religion, socioeconomic variables, sexual preference, gender, belief systems, age, familial status, geographic area, rural/urban distinctions, disability, differences in the type of "intelligences" possessed by various workers, health status, psychological profile, social skills, personality type, dressing style, marital status, and/or numerous other variables. For example, breastfeeding women in a workplace can be included in this definition of cultural diversity. Single parents, gender identity, military or veteran status, and other subgroup status may also be included within the definition of diversity. Accordingly, administrators and managers in virtually all workplaces have now made certain behaviors routine in order to better manage their diverse environments. These activities include practices such as those listed in **BOX 1.9**.

BOX 1.9 Management Practices Toward People Who Are "Different"

- Administrators and managers endanger their organizations if they do not research and learn federal, state, and local laws regarding the management of cultural diversity in their workplaces.
- Not only must administrators and managers know legislative laws that have been proposed or enacted at the federal, state, and local level, their effectiveness can be enhanced by knowing case law that is relevant to their unique workplace.
- Administrators and managers also must assist in creating a culture of acceptance toward differences in the workplace. This is often done by implementing measures to ensure that all labor force participants in the organization are educated regarding that which is tolerable and those behaviors that will result in immediate termination if such actions occur within the workplace and/or at any workplace-sponsored event.
- The organizational attitudes toward diverse groups and subgroups are often reflected in a system of sanctions for those who violate the written and/or unwritten culture of respect.
- Workplaces also establish and educate their employees regarding the steps and processes for reporting behaviors and actions that reflect the dehumanization and the demeaning of members of a specific subgroup.
- The administrators and managers in workplaces also monitor the environment after diversity-related complaints have been filed to ensure that no retaliation occurs.

(continues)

BOX 1.9 Management Practices Toward People Who Are "Different"   *(continued)*

- Administrators and managers conduct comprehensive and honest investigations and seek legal counsel when needed so that the organization, as well as its employees are "protected."
- Administrators, managers, and workplaces also seek to prevent occurrences of complaints by bringing in companies, consultants, and/or utilizing in-house entities to provide diversity and/or other training.
- Many workplaces, in order to support diversity, continually monitor of their organizational structure to ensure that neither individual nor system-based mechanisms are operative that unfairly impact any subgroup.

While such measures as listed in Box 1.9 are used in all workplaces, when healthcare workplaces become the foci of discussion, the burden of managing cultural diversity becomes even more complex because of the various combinations and permutations of intersectionalities that may be operative.

Yet, healthcare workplaces may have a built-in advantage. This is because healthcare administrators, clinicians, and public health professionals can easily use knowledge of health care in general, as well as their familiarity with behavioral health to reframe approaches to the maximization of outcomes in workplaces characterized by diversity. Healthcare administrators and managers have access to research and data from multiple disciplines to unravel the nature of the mechanisms that generate problems in their diverse workplaces. Moreover, healthcare administrators and managers, public health professionals, clinicians, and healthcare institutions are vulnerable to significant losses when diversity management problems impede output maximization. While organizations in other industries may lose profits when issues of diversity affect performance, healthcare institutions are also at risk of losing and/or damaging human lives. Accordingly, over the next few chapters, the nature and causes of various Isms in healthcare workplaces are analyzed within the framework of the *Theory of Central Tendencyism* (a theory that helps explain why some people respond to individuals and groups in the workplace through behavioral incivilities). Additionally, less common workplace "Isms" are discussed and analyzed. As a result of this process, new strategies of reconciliation and remediation are then proposed.

▶ Summary

This chapter provides an overview of data and concepts on the operation of various adverse beliefs, attitudes, and behaviors that exist in workplaces. These forces are called "Isms." Because these Isms often occur simultaneously, we apply the term "intersectionalities" to refer to the interactive nature of these adverse beliefs. This chapter also introduces a brief history which demonstrates that cultural conflict is a natural human phenomenon that occurs when diverse humans come together in common geographical, social, and/or business/economic workplaces. These behaviors are neither condemned nor critiqued. Rather, the task for the healthcare manager and/or human resources manager is to identify solutions that can maximize output in culturally diverse healthcare workplaces before such beliefs, attitudes, and behaviors transform into a workplace characterized by reduced output. Stated differently, the text analyzes the operation of **Diversitism**.

Wrap-Up

Review Questions

1. Based on the data and interpretive bullets discussed in this chapter, develop a PowerPoint presentation that uses your own research to identify and present an "Ism" not discussed in this chapter that may also be present in healthcare workplaces.
2. Have you ever encountered any of the Isms described in this chapter? If so, how did you respond?
3. As a prospective and/or current healthcare manager or administrator, do you have any unique measures you would implement to reduce such forces and prevent losses in the area of output?

Key Terms and Concepts

Ableism

Ageism

Diversitism

Isms

Linguicism

Lookism

Micro-aggression

Micro-assault

Micro-insult

Micro-invalidation

Nameism

Sectarianism

Structural Unemployment

Workplace Isms

References

2020 Census Questions: Race. retrieved from https://2020census.gov/en/about-questions/2020-census-questions-race.html

Achenbaum, W. A. (2014). Robert N. Butler, MD (January 21, 1927–July 4, 2010): Visionary leader. *Gerontologist, 54*(1), 6–12.

Acholonu, R., Mangurian, C., & Linos, E. (2019). TIME's UP Healthcare: Can we put an end to gender inequality and harassment in medicine? *British Medical Journal, 364*, doi:10.1136/bmj.l1987

Alzughaibi, F. (2015). Irish immigration to America: An analysis of the social and economic issues Irish immigrants experienced as conveyed through Toibin's book *Brooklyn*. *American Research Journal of English and Literature, 1*(6).

American Hospital Association, Institute for Diversity in Health Management and Health Research Educational Trust. (2014). 2013 Diversity and disparities: A benchmark study of U.S. Hospitals. https://www.aha.org/ahahret-guides/2014-06-17-2013-diversity-and-disparities-benchmark-study-us-hospitals

American Name Society: Promoting the study of onomastics. *NAMES: A Journal of Onomastics*, https://www.americannamesociety.org/the-journal/

Anand, R., & Winters, M. F. (2008). A Retrospective view of corporate diversity training from 1964 to the present, *Academy of Management Learning & Education, 7*(3), 356–372.

Asian American Coalition for Education (2017). Discrimination in College Admissions, http://asianamericanforeducation.org.

Bar-David, S. (2018). What's in an eye roll? It is time we explore the role of workplace incivility in healthcare. *Israel Journal of Health Policy Research, 7*(1):15. doi:10.1186/s13584-018-0209-0

Berger, P. L. (1954). The sociological study of sectarianism. *Social Research, 21*(4), 467–485.

Bitner, M. J. (1992). Servicescapes: The impact of physical surroundings on customers and employees. *Journal of Marketing, 56*(2), 57–71.

Boston College, Mission & History, https://www.bc.edu/bc-web/about/mission.html

Brewster, K. L., & Rindfuss, R. R. (2000). Fertility and women's employment in industrialized nations. *Annual Review of Sociology, 26*(1), 271–296.

Brophy, J. T., Keith, M. M., & Hurley, M. (2018). Assaulted and unheard: Violence against healthcare staff. *New Solutions. A Journal of Environmental and Occupational Health Policy, 27*(4), 581–606.

Bursell, M. (2007). What's in a name? A field experiment test for the existence of ethnic discrimination in the hiring process. Working Paper 2007-7. Stockholm University Linnaeus Center for Integration Studies. http://www.temaasyl.se/Documents/Forskning /Forskningsstudier/What%E2%80%99s%20in%20a%20name.pdf

Butler, R. N. (1969). Age-ism: Another form of bigotry. *The Gerontologist, 9*(4), 243–246. doi:10.1093/geront/9.4_part_1.243

California Legislative Information. Senate Bill 188 Discrimination: hairstyles. https://leginfo .legislature.ca.gov/faces/billTextClient.xhtml?bill_id=201920200SB188

Call, M. L., Nyberg, A. J., Ployhart, R. E., & Weekley, J. A. (2014). The dynamic nature of collective turnover and unit performance: The impact of time, quality, and replacements. *The Academy of Management Journal, 58*(4). Articles Published Online: 11 Nov 2014 doi:10.5465/amj .2013.0669

Cambridge English Dictionary. Ism. https://dictionary.cambridge.org/us/dictionary/english/ism Retrieved June 20, 2019.

Chandler, P. J., Chandler, C., & Dabbs, M. L. (2000). Provider gender preference in obstetrics and gynecology: A military population. *Military Medicine, 165*(12), 938–940.

Chen, Y. (2012). Dictionary Use and Vocabulary Learning in the Context of Reading. *International Journal of Lexicography, 25*(2), 216–247. doi:10/1093/ij/ecr031

Cherney, J. L. (2011). The rhetoric of ableism, *Disability Studies Quarterly, 31*(3).

Choi, S. H., & Lee, H. (2017). Workplace violence against nurses in Korea and its impact on professional quality of life and turnover intention. *Journal of Nursing Management, 25*(7), 508–518. doi:10.1111/jonm.12488

Cohen, M., Jeanmonod, D., Stankewicz, H., Habeeb, K., Berrios, M., & Jeanmonod, R. (2018). An observational study of patients' attitudes to tattoos and piercings on their physicians: the ART study. *Emergency Medicine Journal, 35*(9), 538–543. doi:10.1136/emermed-2017-206887

Collier, S., Burston, B., & Rhodes, A. (2016). Teaching STEM as a second language. *Journal for Multicultural Education, 10*(3), 257–273.

Collins Dictionary. Ism. https://www.collinsdictionary.com/us/dictionary/english/ism_1. Retrieved June 20, 2019.

Coombs, A. A. T., & King, R. K. (2005). Workplace discrimination: Experience of practicing physicians. *Journal of the National Medical Association, 94*(4), 467–477.

Cydulka, R. K., D'Onofrio, G., Schneider, S., Emerman, C. L., & Sullivan, L. M. (2000). Women in academic emergency medicine. *Academic Emergency Medicine, 7*(9), 999–1007.

Daldy, B., Poot, J., & Roskruge, M. (2013). Perception of workplace discrimination among immigrants and native born New Zealanders IZA DP No. 7504 July 2013, *Discussion Paper No. 7504.*

Dennis, H., & Thomas, K. (2007). Ageism in the workplace. *Generations, 31*(1), 84–89.

Dictionary.com. –ism. https://www.dictionary.com/browse/ism Retrieved June 20, 2019.

Drazewski, P. (2013). Tattoo stigma and job discrimination. Theses and dissertations. *Paper 148.*

EEOC (2018). Age Discrimination in Employment Act (Charges filed with EEOC) (Includes concurrent charges with Title VII, ADA, EPA, and GINA) FY 1997 - FY 2019. https://www .eeoc.gov/eeoc/statistics/enforcement/adea.cfm

English Oxford Dictionaries. ism. https://www.lexico.com/en/definition/ism Retrieved June 20, 2019.

Equal Employment Opportunity Commission. (2019). Memorial Healthcare to pay $74,418 to settle EEOC religious discrimination lawsuit. Press Release. June 25, 2019. https://www.eeoc.gov /eeoc/newsroom/release/6-25-19c.cfm

Equal Employment Opportunity Commission. Montrose Memorial Hospital to pay $400,000 to settle EEOC age discrimination lawsuit. Press Release. January 4, 2018. https://www.eeoc.gov /eeoc/newsroom/release/1-4-18.cfm

European Network Against Racism (2018). Press Release: No progress in curbing racial discrimination in the European labour market – in particular for women of colour. https:// www.enar-eu.org/No-progress-in-curbing-racial-discrimination-in-the-European-labour -market-in-1490

Fasbender, U., & Wang, M. (2016). Negative attitudes toward older workers and hiring decisions: Testing the moderating role of decision makers' core self-evaluations, *Frontiers in Psychology*, 7L2057, doi:10.3389/fpsyg.2016.02057

Fennema, K., Meyer, D. L., & Owen, N. (1990). Sex of physician: patients' preferences and stereotypes. *The Journal of Family Practice, 30*(4), 441–446.

Fougeyrollas, P., & Beauregard, L. (2001). Disability: An interactive person-environment social creation. In: G. L. Albrecht, K. D. Seelman, & M. Bury (Eds). *Handbook of disability studies*. Sage Publications; Thousand Oaks, CA: (pp. 171–194).

Free Dictionary. ism. https://www.thefreedictionary.com/ism Retrieved June 20, 2019.

Freedman, J. (2010). Women in medicine: Are we "there" yet? https://www.medscape.com /viewarticle/732197

French, M., Mortensen, K., & Timming, A. R. (2019). Are tattoos associated with employment and wage discrimination? Analyzing the relationship between body art and labor market outcomes. *Human Relations, 72*, 962–987.

Friedman, E. (2014). U.S. Hospitals and the Civil Rights Act of 1964, Hospitals & Health Networks, https://www.hhnmag.com, Retrieved May 28, 2010.

Gallie, D. (2019). Research on work values in a changing economic and social context. *The Annals of American Academy of Political and Social Science*, 682:1, 26–42. doi:10.1170 /0002716219826038

Gates, D. M. (2004). The Epidemic of violence against healthcare workers. *Occupational and Environmental Medicine, 61*(8), 649–650. doi:10.1136/oem.2004.011548

Gehring, S. (2017). Tragic health care discrimination case sheds light on the future of anti-discrimination measures. National Center for Transgender Equality, https://transequality.org, Accessed, October 6, 2017.

Gerberich, S. G., Church, T. R., McGovern, P. M., Hansen, H. E., Nachreiner, N. M., Geisser, M. S., … Watt, G. D. (2004). An epidemiological study of the magnitude and consequences of work related violence: the Minnesota Nurses' Study. *Occupational and Environmental Medicine, 61*(6), 495–503. doi:10.1136/oem.2003.00729

Goering, S. (2015). Rethinking disability: The social model of disability and chronic disease. *Current Reviews in Musculoskeletal Medicine, 8*(2), 134–138. doi:10.1007/s12178-015-9273

Greene, J., Hibbard, J. H., & Sacks, R. M. (2018). Does the race/ethnicity or gender of a physician's name impact patient selection of the physician? *Journal of the National Medical Association, 110*(3), 206–211.

Gringeri, C. (2019). Book Review: On gender, labor and Inequality. *Affilia, 34*(1), 135–136. doi:10.1177 /0886109918770789

Hamilton, H. (2012). The efficacy of dictionary use while reading for learning new words. *American Annals of the Deaf, 157*(4), 358–372.

Heaton, C. J., & Marquez, J. T. (1990). Patient preference for physician gender in the male genital /rectal exam. *Family Practice Research Journal, 10*(2), 105–115.

Hedegaard, M. S., & Tyran, J-R (2018). The price of prejudice. *American Economic Journal: Applied Economics, 10*(1), 40–63. doi:10.1257/app.20150241

Heejung, C., & Mau, S. (2014). Subjective insecurity and the role of institutions. *Journal of European Social Policy, 24*(4), 303–318. doi:10.1177/0958928714538214

Henegham, S. M. (2012). Employment discrimination faced by the immigration worker – a lesson from the United States and South Africa. *Fordham International Law Journal, 35*(6), Article 4, 1781–1820.

Herring, C. (2009). Does diversity pay? Race, gender, and the business case for diversity. *American Sociological Review, 74*(2), 208–224. doi:10.1177/000312240907400203

Himes, M. (2016). Prejudice against ethnic-sounding names forces people to choose between their identities and success. Quartz. https://qz.com/787189/nyc-chelsea-bomber-name-prejudic e-against-ethnic-sounding-names-forces-people-to-question-their-identities/

Hoeber, F. W. (2001). Drama in the courtroom, theater in the streets: Philadelphia's Irish Riot of 1831. *Pennsylvania Magazine of History and Biography, 125*(3).

Houston, N. A., Secrest, A. M., Harris, R. J., Mori, W. S., Eliason, M. J., Phillips, C. M., & Ferris, L. K. Patient preferences during skin cancer screening examination. (2016). *JAMA Dermatology, 152*(9), 1052–1054.

Howard, J. (2016). Racism in medicine: An "open secret," CNN, cnn.com, Accessed May 28, 2019.

Hsu, I. C., & Lawler, J. J. (2019). An investigation of the relationship between gender composition and organizational performance in Taiwan—The role of task complexity. *Asia Pacific Journal of Management, 36*(1), 275–304.

Huraib, S. B., Nahas, N. A., Al-Balbeesi, H. O., Abu-Aljadayl, F. M., Vellappally, S., & Sukumaran, A. (2015). Patients preferences in selecting a dentist: Survey results from the urban population of Riyadh, Saudi Arabia. *Journal of Contemporary Dental Practice, 16*(3), 201–204.

Joshi, S. C., & Joshi, R. (2018). Doctor becomes a patient: A qualitative study of health care work place violence related perception among junior doctors working in a teaching hospital in India. *International Journal of Community Medicine and Public Health, 5*(5), 1775–1786. doi:10.18203/2394-6040.ijcmph20181381

Kavilanz, P. (2018). The gender pay gap for women doctors is big – and getting worse. Money.cnn .com, Accessed May 14, 2018.

Kim, S. O., Kang, T. W., & Kwon, D. Gender preferences for urologists: Women prefer female urologists. *Urology Journal, 14*(2), 3018–3022.

Konings, J., & Vanormeligen, S. (2015). The impact of training on productivity and wages: Firm-level evidence. *Review of Economics and Statistics, 97*(2), 485–497. doi:10.1162/REST_a_00460

Kydd, A., & Fleming, A. (2015). Ageism and age discrimination in health care: Fact or fiction? A narrative review of the literature. *Maturitas, 81*(4), 432–438.

Lee, H., Ahn, R., Kim, T. H., & Han, E. (2019). Impact of obesity on employment and wages among young adults: Observational study with panel data. *International Journal of Environmental Research and Public Health, 16*(1), 139; doi:10.3390/ijerph16010139

Lee, H., Son, I., Yoon, J., & Kim, S-S (2017). Lookism hurts: Appearance discrimination and self-rated health in South Korea. *International Journal of Equity and Health, 16*(1):204. doi:10.1180 /s12939-017-0678-8

Li, N., Zhang, L., Xiao, G., Chen, J., & Lu, Q. (2019). The relationship between workplace violence, job satisfaction and turnover intention in emergency nurses. *International Emergency Nursing, 45*, 50–55. doi:10.1016/j.ienj.2019.02.007

Library of Congress. Immigration…. https://www.loc.gov/teachers/classroommaterials/presentation sandactivities/presentations/immigration/chinese10.html Accessed July 4, 2019.

Lind, D. (2015). Why Historians Are Fighting About "No Irish Need Apply" Signs — And Why It Matters. Vox.com, Accessed Aug 4, 2015.

Macmillan Dictionary. Ism. https://www.macmillandictionary.com/us/dictionary/american/ism Retrieved June 20, 2019.

Makary, M. A., & Daniel, M. (2016). Medical error–The third leading cause of death in the US. *The British Medical Journal*, 353, i2139, doi:10.1136/bmj.i2139

Mann, C. (2018). Violence against nurses. *The Kansas Nurse, 93*(1), 14–17. www.ksnurses.com.

Maroto, M., Pennenecchio, D., & Patterson, A. C. (2019). Hierarchies of categorical disadvantage: Economic insecurity at the intersection of disability, gender, and race. *Gender & Society, 33*(1), 64–93.

Marušić, A. (2016). What's in a name? The problem of authors' names in research articles, *Biochemia Medica, 26*(2), 174–175. doi:10.11613/B.M.2016.018

Matthew, D. B. (2015). Legal battles against discrimination in healthcare. The Oxford Handbook of U.S. Health Law, *Edited by I. Glenn Cohen, Allison K. Hoffman, and William M. Sage*, Jan 2017, 10.1093/oxfordhb/9780199366521.013.9

Menees, S. B., Inadomi, J. M., Korsnes, S., & Elta, G. H. (2005). Women patients' preference for women physicians is a barrier to colon cancer screening. *Gastrointestinal Endoscopy, 62*(2), 219–223.

Merriam-Webster Dictionary. ism. https://www.merriam-webster.com/dictionary/ism Retrieved June 20, 2019.

Mikkonen, K., Elo, S., Kuivila, H. M., Tuomikoski, A. M., & Kääriäinen, M. (2016). Culturally and linguistically diverse healthcare students' experiences of learning in a clinical environment: A systematic review of qualitative studies. *International Journal of Nursing Studies, 54,* 173–187. doi:10.1016/j.ijnurstu.2015.06.004

Molnar, A. (2010). History of Italian immigration. (from Europe to America: Immigration through family tales). Mount Holyoke. https://www.mtholyoke.edu/~molna22a/classweb/politics /Italianhistory.html

Moore, J., & Continelli, T. (2016). Racial/ethnic pay disparities among registered nurses (RNs) in U.S. hospitals: An econometric regression decomposition. *Health Services Research Journal, 51*(2), 511–29. doi:10.1111/1475-6773.12337. Epub 2016 Mar 1.

Oliver M. The politics of disablement: A sociological approach. St. Martin's Press; New York: 1990.

Oyez. Saint Francis College V. Al-Khazraji. June 23, 2018, www.oyez.org/cases/1986/85-2169.

Paul-Emile, K., Smith, A. K., Lo, B., & Fernández, A. (2016). Dealing with racist patients, *New England Journal of Medicine, 374*(8), 708–711. doi:10.1056/NEJMp1514939

Pedriana, N., & Stryker, R. (2004). The strength of a weak agency: enforcement of Title VII of the 1964 Civil Rights Act and the Expansion of State Capacity, 1965–1971. *American Journal of Sociology, 110*(3), 709–760, The University of Chicago Press, doi:10.1086/422588, http://www .jstor.org/stable/10.1086/422588

Peffer, G. A. Forbidden families: Emigration experiences of Chinese women under the Page Law, 1875–1882. *Journal of American Ethnic History, 6*(1) (Fall 1986), 28–46.

Phillip, J. P. (2016). Workplace violence against health care workers in the United States. *New England Journal of Medicine, 374,* 1661–1669. doi:10.1056/NEJMra1501998

Phillips, K. (2017). Asian American doctor: White nationalist patients refused my care over race. *The Washington Post,* August 21, 2017.

Pingitore, R., Dagoni, B. L., Tindale, R. S., & Spring, B. (1994). Bias against overweight job applicants in a simulated employment interview. *Journal of Applied Psychology, 79*(6), 909–917. doi:10 .103710021-9010,79.6.909

Plunkert, L. M. (1990). The 1980's: A decade of job growth and industry shifts. *Monthly Labor Review, 113*(9), 3–16. https://www.jstor.org/stable/41843521

Rege, A. (2018). Nurse wins $3.83M racial discrimination lawsuit against Hawaii hospital. *Becker's Hospital Review.*

Reynolds, K. L., Cowden, J. D., Brosco, J. P., & Lantos, J. D. (2015). When a family requests a white doctor. *Pediatrics, 136*(2), 381–386.

Robert Wood Johnson Foundation (November 2017). Discrimination in America: Experiences and views of Asian Americans, Harvard, T.H. Chan School of Public Health.

Rosenfeld, P. (2007). Workplace practices for retaining older hospital nurses: Implications from a Study of Nurses with eldercare responsibilities. *Policy, Politics & Nursing Practice, 8*(2), 120–129. doi:10.1177/1527154407303497

Roth, S. (2019). Linguistic capital and inequality to aid relations. *Sociological Research Online, 24*(1), 38–54.

Rubery, J. (2019). The founding of the *Gender, Work and Organization* journal: Reflections 25 Years On. *Gender, Work and Organization, 26*(1), 9–17. doi:10.1111/gwao.12330

Sánchez Ramos, M. (2005). Research on dictionary use by trainee translators, *Translation Journal, 9*(2), https://translation journal.net, Accessed, Wednesday, June 5, 2019.

Schroth, S. J. R. (2008). Fordham: A history and memoir, Revised Edition. Fordham University, ISBN-13: 978-0823229772. OCLC7276145703

Science News (Daily, 2015). New study finds nearly half of American muslim doctors feel scrutinized on the job. https://www.sciencedaily.com. December 11, 2015.

Shamrani, H. A cross-sectional survey of women's provider gender preferences for gynecology and obstetrics care at King Abdulaziz University Hospital. (2016). *Journal of Women's Health Care, 5*(6).

Siklossy, G. Senior Commonwealth Press Officer, (2018). No progress in curbing racial discrimination in the European labour market – In particular for women of color. Press Release by the European Network Against Racism.

Skutnabb-Kangas, T. (2000). Linguistic genocide in education – or worldwide diversity and human rights? Mahwah, NJ & London, UK: Lawrence Erlbaum Associates.

Smith, D. B. (1988). The racial segregation of hospital care revisited: Medicare discharge patterns and their implications. *American Journal of Public Health, 88*(3), 461–463.

Spetz, J. (2016). The nursing profession, diversity, and wages. *Health Services Research, 51*(2), 505–510. doi:10.1111/1475-6773.12476. Epub 2016 Mar 1.

Sue, D. W., Capodilupo, C. M., Torino, G. C., Bucceri, J. M., Holder, A. M., Nadal, K. L., & Esquilin, M. (2007). Racial microaggressions in everyday life: Implications for clinical practice. *The American Psychologist, 62*(4), 271–286.

Symons, X. (2018). Lookism, and what we should do about it, *BioEdge*, https://www.bioedge.org, Retrieved June 3, 2019.

Teaching for Diversity and Social Justice. (2007). History of racism and immigration time line: Key events in the struggle for racial equality in the United States. M. Adams, L. A. Bell, & P. Griffin, (Eds.). Second Ed., Routledge. http://www.racialequitytools.org/resourcefiles/racismmimmigration-timeline.pdf

Tobler, K. J., Wu, J., Ayatallah, M., Pier, B., Torrealday, S., & Londra, L. (2016). Gender preference of the obstetrician gynecologist provider: A systematic review and meta-analysis. *Obstetrics and Gynecology, 127*, 43S.

Toossi, M. (2002). A century of change: The U.S. labor force, 1950-2050. U.S. Department of Labor, Bureau of Labor Statistics. *Monthly Labor Review, 125*(5), 15–28. doi:10.2307/41845363

U.S. Bureau of Census (2010). DP-1 Profile of General Population and Housing Characteristics: 2010 Demographic Profile Data. United States Census Bureau. Retrieved June 20, 2019.

U.S. Bureau of Census (2010). DP-02 Selected social characteristics in the United States – 2006-2010 American community survey, 5-year estimates. *United States Census Bureau*. Retrieved June 20, 2019.

U.S. Bureau of the Census (2004). Ancestry: 2000. Census 2000 Brief. Pg. 8. https://www.census.gov/history/pdf/ancestry.pdf

U.S. Bureau of Census. U.S. Census Bureau. ACS Demographic and Housing Estimates. 2018 ACS i-Year Estimates Data Profiles. Table DP05. https://data.census.gov/cedsci/table?q=race%20ethnicity%20in%202018&hidePreview=false&tid=ACSDP1Y2018.DP05&t=Race%20and%20Ethnicity&y=2018&vintage=2018

U.S. Bureau of Census. U.S. Census Bureau. 2018 Estimate Comparative Social Characteristics in the United States. 2018 ACS 1-Year Estimates Comparison Profiles. Table CP02. https://data.census.gov/cedsci/table?q=CP02&tid=ACSCP1Y2018.CP02&vintage=2018

U.S. Bureau of the Census (2019). U.S. and World Population Clock. https://www.census.gov/popclock/ Accessed August 1, 2019.

United States Department of Labor, Bureau of Labor Statistics, Database Tables and Calculations, Labor Force Statistics from the Current Population Survey, series I.D.: LnU04000000. Unemployment Rate, Percent or rate 16 years and over 1947–2017, Data extended on May 2018 (12:1925 pm)

U.S. Department of Labor, Bureau of Labor Statistics (2017). Table 11. Employed persons by detailed occupation, sex, race, and Hispanic or Latino ethnicity. https://www.bls.gov/cps/aa2017/cpsaat11.pdf

U.S. Department of Labor, Bureau of Labor Statistics (2017). Table 18. Employed persons by detailed industry, sex, race, and Hispanic or Latino ethnicity. https://www.bls.gov/cps/aa2017/cpsaat18.pdf

U.S. Department of Labor, Bureau of Labor Statistics (2018). Table 11. Employed persons by detailed occupation, sex, race, and Hispanic or Latino ethnicity. https://www.bls.gov/cps/cpsaat11.pdf

U.S. Department of Labor, Bureau of Labor Statistics (2018). Table 18. Employed persons by detailed industry, sex, race, and Hispanic or Latino ethnicity at https://www.bls.gov/cps/cpsaat18.pdf

U.S. Department of Labor, Occupational Safety and Health Administration publication, Workplace Violence in Healthcare: Understanding the Challenge, (2015). https://www.osha.gov/Publications/OSHA3826.pdf

Van Ness, C. J., & Lynch, D. A. (2000). Male adolescents and physician sex preference. *Archives of Pediatrics & Adolescent Medicine, 154*(1), 49–53.

Van Ryn, M., Hardeman, R., Phelan, S. M., Burgess, D. J., Dovidio, J. F., Herrin, J., Burke, S. E., Nelson, D. B., Perry, S., Yeazel, M., & Przedworski, J. M. (2015). Medical school experiences associated with change in implicit racial bias among 3547 students: A medical student CHANGES Study Report. *Journal of General Internal Medicine, 30*(12), 1748–56. doi:10.1007/s11606-015-3447-7. Epub 2015 Jul 1.

Wang, L. W. (2018). 2020 Census to keep racial, ethnic categories used in 2010. National Public Radio. https://www.npr.org/2018/01/26/580865378/census-request-suggests-no-race-ethnicity -data-changes-in-2020-experts-say

Whalen, W. J. (1981). Minority religions in America. Alba House.

Whitgob, E. E., Blankenburg, R. L., & Bogetz, A. L. (2016). The discriminatory patient and family: Strategies to address discrimination towards trainees. *Academic Medicine, 91*(11 Association of American Medical Colleges Learn Serve Lead: Proceedings of the 55th Annual Research in Medical Education Sessions):S64–S69.

Wong, A. H., Ray, J. M., & Iennaco, J. D. (2019). Workplace violence in health care and agitation management: Safety for patients and health care professionals are two sides of the same coin. *The Joint Commission Journal on Quality Patient Safety, 45*(2), 71–73.

Wright, P., Ferris, S. P., Hiller, J. S., & Kroll, M. (2017). Competitiveness through management of diversity: Effects on stock price valuation, *Academy of Management Journal, 38*(1). doi:10.5465/256736

Wyman, M. F., Shiovitz-Ezra, S., & Bengel, J. (2018). Ageism in the health care system: Providers, patients, and systems. *Contemporary Perspectives on Ageism*, 193–212. doi:10.1007/978-3-319 -73820-8_13

Young, A., Chaudry, H. J., Pei, X., Arnhart, K., Dugan, M., and Snyder, G. B. (2017). A census of actively licensed physicians in the United States, 2016. *Journal of Medical Regulation, 103*(2), 7–21.

Zhang, X., & Zheng, Y. (2019). Gender differences in self-view and desired salaries: A study on online recruitment website users in China. *PloS One, 14*(1), e0210072. doi:10.1371/journal .pone.0210072

Zinn, H. (1990). *A People's History of the United States.* 154–155. Harper Perennial Modern Classics: NY. ISBN-13: 978-0060838652

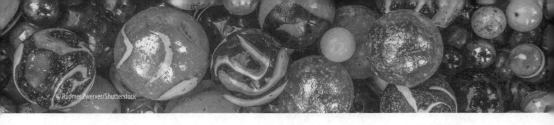

CHAPTER 2

What Is Central Tendencyism and How Does It Affect Healthcare and Other Workplaces?

"People fail to get along because they fear each other; they fear each other because they don't know each other; they don't know each other because they have not communicated with each other."

– Martin Luther King, Jr

LEARNING OBJECTIVES

After completing this chapter, each reader will be able to:

- Define output maximization.
- Describe how Central Tendency can relate to adverse beliefs, attitudes, and behaviors about people who are statistical outliers from the "norm."
- Define and identify implicit bias.
- Summarize research regarding the magnitude of "undesirable behaviors" in the workplace.
- Discuss Central Tendencyism as a framework for understanding how it serves as the basis of "Isms."
- Analyze the linkages between Central Tendencyism and "uncivil" behaviors.

▶ Introduction: Human Behavior and Healthcare Workplaces

Despite the underdiscussion of Psychology and Sociology in healthcare administration, human behavior forms the very foundation of the jobs of healthcare senior, middle, and first-level managers. A closer look at position descriptions of healthcare administrators and managers reveals the vast responsibilities that these positions involve. In addition to planning, organizing, directing, and controlling human and nonhuman resources to support health services, these essential organizational entities must also maximize output. *Output maximization* is the production of the largest amount and highest-quality of output possible from available human and nonhuman resources. Output maximization requires a high level of skills in capital budgeting and/or in using single or multiple channel models for sourcing a healthcare organization's supplies. But, output maximization involves competencies beyond those taught in general healthcare management and/or human resource management courses. Specifically, output maximization cannot occur without harmonious and synchronized interactions between workers within a healthcare and/or non-healthcare environment. Accordingly, individual and subgroup "Isms" can create behaviors and interactions that result in decreased productivity. In a review and analysis of more than 12,482 studies, Tricco et al. (2018) found that bullying, sexual harassment, verbal hostility, threats against continued employment, and/or career advancement, and other examples of underdeveloped humanism were all present in healthcare workplaces. **Underdeveloped humanism** refers to persons with insufficient empathy for others who are "in" need.

Workers who engage in underdeveloped humanisms toward others are not the exception. Numerous workers in the studies analyzed by Tricco et al. (2018) had experienced adverse attitudes, beliefs, and behaviors. While the study included private companies, public administration workplaces, and all levels of educational institutions, approximately 47.83% of the studies identified were specific to healthcare workplaces. Approximately 20 or 86.96% of the 23 studies included a more detailed analysis of healthcare workplaces. Some analysts would argue that workplace practices that violate workers' overall humanity are societal and not merely organizational. This may be true since the workers who displayed the negative beliefs, attitudes and behaviors as described by Tricco et al. (2018) included upper management executives, middle managers, general workers, and contractors.

Accordingly, it is imperative that healthcare administrators and managers perform an analysis and implement measures that will facilitate change. A critical examination of Tricco et al.'s (2008) research suggests that further analysis is needed before effective strategies of remediation can be designed and implemented. For example, approximately 91.3% of the interventions used in these prior studies, although focused on the individual, involved only *one training session* to correct adverse output-diminishing workplace behaviors. Accordingly, it is not surprising that the results of the approach were primarily a change in awareness. ***Absolutely no changes in work behaviors occurred.***

Other studies have also identified healthcare workplaces as sources of behaviors that are counterproductive to increased output. Students, residents, and faculty have provided evidence of exposure to negative treatment by specialists and other physicians with greater levels of **achieved power** or power that develops through one's own efforts. Phillips et al. (2018) label such behaviors as problems of **incivility** and confirm that nurses and other personnel in healthcare workplaces experience incivilities.

Shuck et al. (2018) suggest that new behavioral theories are necessary to generate new solutions to such counterproductive behaviors. For example, some evidence exists suggesting that information that is learned in training workshops is not always applied correctly. Other initiatives have also been tested. One approach to change negative behavior that has been used is called reinforcement theory. **Reinforcement theory** is, of course, not new. Winokur (1971) provided an overview of this classic theory. Reinforcement theory stemmed from the work of B. F. Skinner who introduced the notion of operant conditioning (Skinner, 1938). Building upon the research of Pavlov (Windholz, 1997) and other psychologists, Skinner conducted experiments that demonstrated how human behavior can be shaped by consistent rewards and punishments. Reinforcement theory showed how behaviors can be influenced by directly following desirable behaviors with rewards and by attaching negative consequences to undesirable behavior.

Accordingly, it is not surprising that reinforcement theory was adopted and applied in healthcare and other workplaces. Wiley (1997), for example, summarizes results from employee surveys for 1946, 1980, 1986, and 1992 regarding the type of rewards used to promote positive workplace behaviors. Because these surveys revealed that money was an effective motivator, many workplaces adopted such a strategy. Specifically, workplaces that used this behavioral theory provided external financial rewards to workers for not displaying negative behaviors and thus impeding productivity. However, reinforcement theory didn't always deliver improvements in productivity. According to Shuck et al. (2018) interventions using financial incentives sometimes results in lower output. Shuck and associates introduced **Self-Determination Theory (SDT)** as a tool for understanding human behavior in the workplace. Self-determination theory is based upon the belief that forces internal to individuals oftentimes drive their behavioral choices. Ryan and Deci (2000) suggest that within the workplace, the social environment can generate responses that are "…proactive and engaged or …passive and alienated," and, as a result, impact the self-determination located in the individual. For example, proactivity and engagement will motivate maximized output.

But, whether the workplace delivers healthcare services and/or another specialty of services, proactivity and engagement will, according to this theory, only occur under three conditions: 1) past and present circumstances must combine to make workers feel competent and empowered to successfully complete their duties; 2) workers must feel in control of their workplace choices and behaviors; and 3) workers must feel an alliance with and a connection to others in the work environment. Thus, this theory moves the focus from the individual to the workplace. In other words, all humans in the workplace must reinforce the three requirements that will support **output maximization**.

Self-determination theory has been previously applied in healthcare workplaces. Patrick and Williams (2012) and Rucker (2000), for example, describe how it has been used in various public health environments. These researchers recommend that this theory be partnered with motivational interviewing in order to foster positive results. However, SDT has been used less frequently in healthcare administration despite the fact that employees who work in healthcare workplaces that are conducive to bullying and other negative behaviors will be unable to achieve increased output. Although self-determination theory can clarify how to enhance output in health care and/or other workplaces despite negative workplace experiences, too little attention has been paid to understanding the impact that negative words and actions in the workplace can have on output. The **Theory of Central Tendencyism** was conceptualized in order to better analyze how "Isms" emerge and prevail in health care and other workplaces. However, before introducing this theory, additional attention must be directed toward "uncivil behaviors" as a barrier to output maximization.

Uncivil Behaviors in the Workplace

The word "uncivil" is a common one in the English language. **BOX 2.1** lists some of the definitions of **uncivil** that were found in various dictionaries. (Once again, definitions from dictionaries have been extracted because these learning tools are the primary instruments for standardizing language.)

As a review of these definitions reveal, the type of rude, unfriendly, abrupt, bad-mannered, discourteous, insulting behaviors that are oftentimes labeled as "discrimination" do, indeed, comprise incivilities. These incivilities may be based on race/ethnicity, nationality, sex, sexual preferences, religious beliefs, income levels, social classes, and/or a myriad of other characteristics. Independently of cause, these incivilities have the power to reduce human output. However, before a healthcare administrator or manager can affect such behaviors, it is necessary to have a clearer understanding of the beliefs that cause these incivilities. This text introduces the *Theory of Central Tendencyism* to clarify some of the forces that operate in health care and other workplaces that reduce output maximization via incivilities.

BOX 2.1 Definitions of Uncivil

- Uncivil—not civilized: barbarous | lacking in courtesy; ill-mannered, impolite | uncivil remarks | not conducive to civil harmony and welfare.
  (Courtesy of Merriam-Webster Dictionary. Uncivil. https://www.merriam-webster.com/dictionary/uncivil?utm_campaign=sd&utm_medium=serp&utm_source=jsonld)
- Uncivil—abrupt; bad-mannered; barbaric; blunt; boorish; coarse; curt; discourteous; gross; gruff; ill-mannered; impolite; inconsiderate; insulting; mannerless; uncivilized; uncouth; uncultured; unfriendly; ungentlemanly; unmannerly; unpolished; unrefined; vulgar.
  ("Uncivil." Merriam-Webster.com Dictionary, Merriam-Webster, https://www.merriam-webster.com/dictionary/uncivil. Accessed 20 Apr. 2020.)

Constructed by the authors from the cited sources.

▶ Introducing…Behavioral Central Tendencyism

Behavioral incivilities occur across subgroups that extend beyond those that are typically associated with "discrimination." As discussed, numerous Isms are operative in America's workplaces and in the workplaces of other countries throughout the world. As previously mentioned, ageism and ableism are two sources of incivilities in health care and other workplaces. However, incivilities related to race/ethnicity and sex are the types of Isms that are most commonly discussed.

Independently of cause, incivilities are observable in educational, political, economic, health care, and numerous other subsystems. As is known, racism, or incivilities based on physical differences, still exist in the United States and in other countries. Racism generates incivilities based on physical characteristics because such differences are easy to perceive. But, not only do individuals engage in uncivil behaviors based on physical differences, institutions also do so. For example, Williams and Rucker (2000) reveal that many current initiatives, guidelines, and policies of institutions may unintentionally encourage bias and stereotyping. As a result, uncivil behaviors may be observable among employees based upon these physical differences. In *Modern Healthcare*, Livingston (2018) links the lack of racial diversity in the "c-suite" personnel of the nation's hospitals and in other healthcare institutions as an outcome of institutional incivilities.

Similarly, as the nation's citizens grow older and the cost of living rises, more people age 55 years or older will choose to remain in the workplace. Yet, in the United States, age 55 is considered as the beginning of the retirement age. This retirement age floor is confirmed by the fact that the Internal Revenue Service enforces a Rule of 55 which permits withdrawals from one's retirement funds if an employee is voluntarily and/or involuntarily terminated after they reach the age of 55 years. However, age, like race or sex, is a visible physical attribute. Thus, ageism absolutely exists in America's workplaces. The Editor-in-Chief of *AARP* (October/November, 2018), in an article entitled, "That Last Acceptable Prejudice?", reveals that their organization's original research based on a 2018 survey of workers found that approximately 61% of those surveyed (age 45 and older) had personally experienced or observed incivilities being directed toward them due to their age (Love, 2018). Yet, only 4% of the respondents indicated that they had ever formally reported these incivilities. Ageism will continue to be operative in the workplaces throughout America given that seniors are a rapidly growing segment of the population. However, not merely workers, but patients in healthcare workplaces also experience ageism that is directed toward them by physicians and other medical professionals. Rogers, et al. (2015), in a study of 6,017 adults with an average age of 67 years, found that approximately 18% of the respondents indicated that they had experienced incivilities by healthcare workers. Such experiences were not benign. These experiences sometimes resulted in new disabilities. Additionally, existing disabilities sometimes became more severe. Such outcomes occurred in approximately 29% of the respondents who had experienced incivilities on a more frequent basis. Similarly, because a person's sex is also visible, sexism is also often discussed.

Isms which exist in healthcare and other workplaces require additional analysis. For example, all Isms generate results that affect output maximization. However, Isms are most often **normatively** discussed.

Our analysis seeks to trace the impact of such behaviors to a more global standard of ethics—the impact on humankind's chances of survival. Central Tendencyism can help explain how Isms operate with a particular focus on Isms that have been previously undiscussed, under-discussed, and/or analytically oversimplified.

For example, Hammer (2017) reported on research that confirms that incivilities are often directed toward people who are "... less attractive." In turn, those considered "attractive" are rewarded for this non–productivity-related characteristic. In other words, lookism is practiced. Some evidence exists that physicians who are "of a certain age" may experience formal and/or informal incivilities because of ageism (Beekman, 2018). *Classism* and *rankism* also operate in workplaces. Ingram (2006) describes how classism and rankism can lead to institutional and/or direct incivilities in the workplace. He explains that healthcare and other workplaces are hierarchical. This can breed work-related incivilities that impede productivity. Specifically, those of higher rank implicitly or explicitly apply beliefs, attitudes, and behaviors that assign lower human value to those of a lower rank. Fuller (2003) indicates that classism and rankism in workplaces assign titles of "somebodies and nobodies" to workers. (Some individuals who have been employed in healthcare workplaces for lengthy periods of time would argue that such hierarchical arrangements are particularly observable in healthcare workplaces.)

The *U.S. News and World Report*, in their 2019 Best Jobs (2019) publication, notes that Americans rank healthcare workplaces as better places for employment than almost all other occupational areas. Yet, even within healthcare institutions, the "somebodies" and "nobodies" segmentation definitely exists (Mathews, 2014). Independent of the exact ranking, a strong hierarchical structure that allows greater incivilities toward people as rank order descends does, indeed, exist in healthcare workplaces.

Independent of the precise Ism that generates the behavior, exposure to incivilities by humans has an adverse effect on their overall life outcomes and on their ability to be productive. Basic civilities can be "awarded" to all humans independent of social and/or occupational position. Yet, it appears that this may not be the case in some healthcare and other workplaces.

For example, the American Nurses Association (July 22, 2015) published a position paper that strongly advocates for the abolition of incivilities in the healthcare workplace. The research specifically mentions the negative behaviors that nurses experience while on the job. Porath and Pearson (2013) specifically address the impact of such behaviors on output maximization. The National Center for Professional & Research Ethics (NCPRE) lists the types of behaviors that are commonly directed toward people of lower ranks. An incivility can be a simple act such as a physician not making eye contact with and/or speaking to a facility maintenance worker in a hallway. A nurse using an annoying or irritated tone with a certified nursing assistant is engaging in an incivility. A hospital administrator who shows anger toward his or her administrative staff is guilty of an incivility. However, people who initiate incivilities can generate an impact in the workplace that incites a reaction. Andersson and Pearson (1999) argue that each incivility in a workplace has the potential to create a chain reaction. Indeed, these authors indicate that once initiated, "starting and tipping" (pg. 452) points will occur among participants in the workplace. Ultimately, the number of incivilities will grow and "secondary spirals" (pg. 452) will result. A viral-like effect can occur within the healthcare and other workplaces. As a result, output maximization can be greatly impacted.

Such reactions appear to be based on scientific laws and principles. Current and/or past students of chemistry may remember stoichiometric calculations involving reactions between the masses of two reactants. When specific quantities of reactants are combined, the use of stoichiometric calculators will reveal that the theoretical yield (or the maximum amount of product that can be produced) will generally exceed the percent yield. Thus, by combining reactants, the overall efficiency of the reaction is decreased. A similar process occurs in the healthcare workplace, thereby creating exponential rather than linear decreases in the overall efficiency of the workplace.

A parallel process is observable in biology that demonstrates how healthcare and other work environments can benefit from diversity. Biologists often hail the element, carbon. Carbon shows the potential positive outcomes that can stem from diversity. This is because it is carbon's molecular diversity that has generated the many life forms that are seen on Earth. Healthcare and other workplaces can achieve a similar effect if adverse reactions to human differences can be changed.

Bar-David (2018) discusses behaviors such as "…belittling comments or dismissive gestures (eye rolling, lip sounds, sighs, muttering, skipping greetings, gossip, social exclusion, silent treatment, sarcasm, and even the rude use of mobile devices" (pg. 15), as demonstrative of productivity-inhibiting behaviors. Klingberg et al. (2018) suggest that productivity-reducing incivilities frequently occur among physicians and other personnel in emergency departments. Fuller-Rowell et al.'s (2018) research leads to the conclusion that the health consequences of a lower economic class that occur over time at the macro-level also has counterparts at the organizational level.

While incivilities in healthcare workplaces can stem from personalities and/or the rank in the organizational structure of the healthcare workplace, these incivilities often reflect subgroup biases. Indeed, the incivilities that exist within a workplace because of subgroup biases are referred to as **cultural diversitisms**.

This term includes cultural behaviors associated with race/ethnicity, sex, sexual preference, country of origin, religion, and other more frequently discussed "Isms" as well as "Isms" that are more uncommon. The Theory of Central Tendencyism provides insights into how incivilities stemming from human differences emerge and become prevalent in healthcare and other workplaces.

▶ Isms, Incivilities, Healthcare Workplaces, and Output Maximization

The Theory of Central Tendencyism is based on the statistical concept of central tendency. Approximately, 7,790,736,575 people inhabited the earth as of Thursday, June 11, 2020 (Worldometers, 2020). Humans use different statistical concepts to describe each individual. Thus, people's oneness is subdivided into related groups so that they can be statistically measured. These measures begin with continents, progress to countries, states, cities, and even smaller divisions. ("Nation" is different from "state" in that nation references the people, their history, and their culture.) Yet, central tendency characterizes each of these social/political concepts.

More specifically, within every group or subgroup, the *implicit* questions are: 1) "What are the mean, median, and/or modal physical and behavioral characteristics of the individuals in the defined group?; and 2) How much can an individual and/or subgroup differ from the average before they are subjected to incivilities"?

All values in the universe of interest cluster around a mean. The **mean** references the "average" of a set of values that is numerically calculated by adding all values and dividing them by the number of values. The arithmetic mean is only useful when it is combined with a measure of dispersion.

Most of the values will differ from the mean. **Dispersion** measures how much these values differ from the mean as a whole. The variance represents how much the values differ from the mean as a total. The standard deviation serves as a measure of the average amount of variance from the mean. Statistics tell us that most values (68%) fall "+" or "−" one standard deviation from the mean. Approximately 27% of the values will fall "+" or "−" two standard deviations from the mean. Only 5% of the values will fall plus or minus three standard deviations from the mean. While some analysts have critiqued the normal curve (Limpert and Stahel, 2011), central tendency and dispersion do provide a conceptual framework that clarifies human behavior in general, and in workplaces. The world is composed of groups and subgroups, each with their own central tendency. This central tendency then shapes expectations when members of these groups are encountered. The expectation of sameness also extends from this concept. In other words, central tendency creates an expectation of a certain degree of "sameness" among and between all humans. As **FIGURE 2.1** demonstrates, multiple "normal curves" with their own central tendencies and standard deviations define various human groups and subgroups.

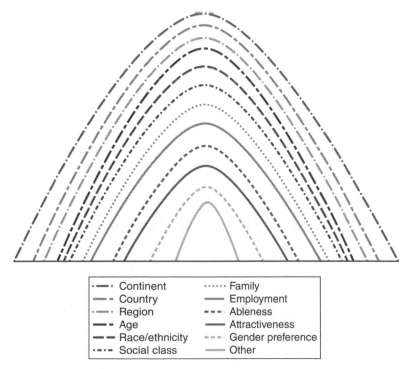

·—· Continent	······ Family
—·– Country	—— Employment
·—·· Region	—-—· Ableness
—·– Age	—— Attractiveness
—— Race/ethnicity	—-—· Gender preference
····- Social class	—— Other

FIGURE 2.1 Groups and subgroups.

Social norms then drive expectations regarding the various groups and subgroups. These measures also define the "average" degree of variation that is "acceptable" for each group or subgroup in each of the above "worlds." Social norms support central tendencyism by utilizing sanctions that reward and/or punish individuals for adherence and/or nonadherence to norms. These group and subgroup norms define an acceptable type of order. This order, to a large degree, dictates behavioral tendencies.

Thus, central **tendency** simply means that other humans develop beliefs, attitudes, behaviors, and norms that target those whose tendencies and/or physical traits deviate from the norm. However, the negative evaluation of those who are different are based on behavioral as well as physical qualities. Common definitions of human "tendencies" can be introduced. These are listed in **BOX 2.2**.

Various groups of humans try to make all people fit the mean for the group. In order to generate a greater "fit" of individual behaviors with the mean behaviors of each group or subgroup, incivilities are directed toward individuals who adopt behaviors and/or who have physical characteristics that are one or more standard deviations from the "central tendencyism" of the group. If the behaviors and/or physical characteristics place them three standard deviations from the mean, the incivilities are even more pronounced. Specifically, other individuals who are within one standard deviation direct incivilities toward people who are two or more standard deviations from the mean. They do this because physical and/or behavioral conformity is more acceptable than nonconformity. Thus, each of these groups promote central tendencyism in order to achieve stability. However, these "norms" can inhibit human growth and development. Moreover, the norms that are generated are not based on an arithmetic mean but on a weighted mean that is calculated.

Stratification emerges and sustains itself through sanctions that, in many instances, include incivilities directed toward individuals and groups who are two to three standard deviations from this weighted mean. Central tendencyism operates within healthcare and other workplaces.

Although terms such as fairness, equity, social justice, and/or other standard concepts are often used to challenge central tendencyism, such normative concepts have not been incorporated into the Theory of Central Tendencyism. Health care and other environments will experience highly successful human relationships and higher levels of productivity in the absence of incivilities. Thus, human behaviors that minimize incivilities are essential to human survival not because of ethics, but

---

BOX 2.2 Definitions of Human "Tendencies"

- Tendency—A likelihood to happen or to have a particular characteristic or effect. (Definition of 'Tendency' from Cambridge Dictionary, www.dictionary.cambridge.org, © Cambridge University Press. Used with permission.)
- Tendency—An inclination, disposition, an attitude of mind especially one that favors one alternative over others; leaning, propensity; A general direction in which something tends to move. (Princeton WordNet. Tendency. http://wordnetweb.princeton.edu/perl/webwn)

Constructed by the authors from the cited sources.

as a result of economic efficiency, a minimally stressful workplace, and the psychic income that accompanies pleasantries.

Although the mean is the most common measure of central tendency, the median defines the "average" as being the "value" that lies in the middle. In society, there are subgroups, patterns of behavior, etc., which personify the "acceptable." Likewise, the mode defines the value with the greatest frequency. Again, these concepts complement central tendencyism based on the mean. Human groups that have the greatest "frequency," even if they are a plurality and not a majority, have greater power. If that power is abused, incivilities may be directed toward other non-modal groups. All definitions of central tendency used in statistics can be seen in human society and may encourage incivilities in human interactions across groups and subgroups.

But, as mentioned, incivilities in society in general, and/or in the workplace, do not support the survival, growth, and development of human beings. Moreover, the changing needs of humans require that "groups," whether 1, 2, or 3 standard deviations from the arithmetic and/or weighted mean, develop over time. Because group members do not understand the need for change which will benefit humans in these new and emerging "presents," Isms occur with incivilities being directed toward those individuals and groups who are two or more standard deviations from the existing norms. Healthcare and other workplaces currently exemplify Central Tendencyism. This book demonstrates this phenomenon by examining only four current Isms—diversitism, sexualism, IQism, and heterosexism. These Isms are defined, demonstrated, and recommendations are made for their resolution. However, the range of Isms in healthcare and/or other workplaces are far more vast than those discussed herein.

▶ Summary

Healthcare workplaces currently hire and sustain numerous workers in the United States. Health care, like education, is a human capital investment industry. Thus, small losses in productivity can multiply in a society. This multiplier effect transcends the impact upon Gross Domestic Product. At this point in time, the future of humankind and all life requires maximum output across all industries. However, because of their roles as "tools of production," healthcare and education in particular must maximize output to support human capital development. However, human survival also depends on strengthening social capital.

Human capital is the entire inventory of information and knowledge, behaviors, creativity, and other aspects of humankind that contribute to the allocation, production, and distribution of the goods and services needed for survival and comfort. But, human capital alone is insufficient. Human survival and development also require that social capital be maximized. Social capital refers to the processes, procedures, activities, and benefits that accrue when humans interact as a group. In such a case, the whole can become greater than the sum of its parts. The people themselves become instruments and tools. They utilize their intellect, emotions, nurturance, creativity, and overall nonphysical assets to support each other. Social and physical capital can maximize all forms of output when they are formed, operated, and sustained within the context of civility. Civility supports the maximization of human interactions. Laws, folkways, mores, and other norms are defined at various points in history to increase and sustain civility among and within human and nonhuman living things. (While the emphasis herein has been output maximization within the workplace, the synergistic relationship among all living things requires that civility be practiced.)

Moreover, the need for civility may possibly be greater now than at any time in the past. Both historically and currently, multiple uncontrollable forces have threatened the survival of living things on earth. Climate and biodiversity and other documented threats do, indeed, suggest that whether current and future threats are equal to, greater than, or less than past threats, humans will benefit if they support civilities that prevent, delay, eliminate, and/or adapt to current and future threats. This handbook is intended to make a small contribution to this imperative by introducing new views and analyses of selected incivility-based "Isms" that inhibit and/or reduce output maximization in healthcare workplaces.

Healthcare administrators and managers work closely with human resources managers to acquire and retain workers who can deliver maximum output at the lowest possible costs. Workplace Isms interfere with these objectives. However, for healthcare administrators and managers to minimize the negative impact of workplace Isms, it is necessary to understand how such forces emerge and operate. This chapter introduced the Theory of Central Tendencyism as a framework for understanding the emergence and operation of the various systems of adverse beliefs, attitudes, and behaviors that assign differential value to healthcare and other workers. This framework—the Theory of Central Tendencyism—is used to analyze only a few of the many Isms that exist. Because the analytical framework used is different, rather unique interventions for healthcare administrators and managers are recommended.

Wrap-Up

Review Questions

1. The term "underdeveloped humanism" is introduced to describe the cause of the incivilities that one worker sometimes directs toward other workers. Have you identified any incivilities among people within your social circle that appear to be related to "underdeveloped humanism"?
2. Output maximization is another term that is defined in this chapter. Based on your knowledge of human resources management, do you, as an individual, maximize output? How can you use your individual human resources to better maximize the outputs you desire in your life?
3. Based on your work on group projects, do most individuals appear to engage in output maximization?
4. Based on your understanding of Central Tendencyism, support or critique the concept.

Key Terms and Concepts

Achieved Power
Cultural Diversitisms
Dispersion
Incivility
Mean
Normatively
Output Maximization

Reinforcement Theory
Self-Determination Theory (SDT)
Tendency
Theory of Central Tendencyism
Uncivil
Underdeveloped Humanisms

References

American Nurses Association (July 22, 2015), American Nurses Association Position Statement on Incivility, Bullying, and Workplace Violence. https://www.nursingworld.org/practice-policy/nursing-excellence/official-position-statements/id/incivility-bullying-and-workplace-violence/

Andersson, L. M., & Pearson, C. M. (1999). Tit for tat? The spiraling effect of incivility in the workplace. *Academy of Management Review, 24*(3), 452–471.

Bar-David, S. (2018). What's in an eye roll? It is time we explore the role of workplace incivility in healthcare. *Israel Journal of Health Policy Research, 7*(1), 15. doi:10.1186/s13584-018-0209-0

Beekman, A. T. F. (2018). Aging affects us all: Aging physicians and screening for impaired professional proficiency. *The American Journal of Geriatric Psychiatry, 26*(6), 641–642.

Cambridge English Dictionary (n.d.) Tendency. https://dictionary.cambridge.org/us/dictionary/english/tendency

Collins English Dictionary (n.d.) uncivil. https://www.collinsdictionary.com/us/dictionary/english/uncivil

Dictionary.com (n.d.) Uncivil. https://www.dictionary.com/browse/uncivil

Dictionary.com (n.d.) Tendency. https://www.dictionary.com/browse/tendency

Free Dictionary (n.d.) Uncivil. https://www.thefreedictionary.com/uncivil

Fuller, R. W. (2003). *Somebodies and Nobodies: Overcoming the Abuse of Rank. Catholic Education. A Journal of Inquiry and Practice, 10*(3), Article 9. https://digitalcommons.lmu.edu/cgi/viewcontent.cgi?referer=https://www.google.com/&httpsredir=1&article=1416&context=ce

Fuller-Rowell, T. E., Curtis, D. S., Chae, D. H., & Ryff, C. D. (2018). Longitudinal health consequences of socioeconomic disadvantage: Examining perceived discrimination as a mediator. *Health Psychology, 37*(5), 491–500.

Hammer, C. (2017). A Look into lookism: An evaluation of discrimination based on physical attractiveness. *Undergraduate Honors Capstone Projects.* 207. Retrieved February 14, 2020, from https://digitalcommons.usu.edu/honors/207

Ingram, P. D. (2006). The ups and downs of the workplace. *Journal of Extension, 44*(3), 5–8.

Klingberg, K., Gadelhak, K., Jegerlehner, S. N., Brown, A. D., Exadaktylos, A. K., & Srivastava, D. S. (2018). Bad manners in the Emergency Department: Incivility among doctors. *PloS One, 13*(3), e0194933.

Limpert, E. & Stahel, W. A. (2011). Problems with using the normal distribution—and ways to improve quality and efficiency of data analysis. *PloS One, 6*(7), e21403. doi:10.1371/journal.pone.0021803

Livingston, S. (2018). Racism still a problem in healthcare's C-suite: Efforts aimed at boosting diversity in healthcare leadership fail to make progress. *Modern Healthcare*, February 24, 2018. https://www.modernhealthcare.com/article/20180224/NEWS/180229948

Love, R. (2018). The last acceptable prejudice. *AARP Magazine, Oct/Nov 2018 Issue, 61*(6B), 4.

Mathews, Z. (2014). Doctor is the World's Most Respected Profession, Kool1079.com. https://kool1079.com/doctor-is-the-worlds-most-respected-profession/

Merriam-Webster Dictionary (n.d.). Uncivil. https://www.merriam-webster.com/dictionary/uncivil?utm_campaign=sd&utm_medium=serp&utm_source=jsonld

Merriam-Webster Dictionary (n.d.). Tendency. https://www.merriam-webster.com/dictionary/tendency

Oxford Dictionary (n.d.). Uncivil. https://www.lexico.com/en/definition/uncivil

Patrick, H., & Williams, G. C. (2012). Self-determination theory: Its application to health behavior and complementarity with motivational interviewing. *The International Journal of Behavioral Nutrition and Physical Activity, 9*(18).

Phillips, G. S., MacKusick, C. I., & Whichello, R. (2018). Workplace incivility in nursing: A literature review through the lens of ethics and spirituality. *Journal of Christian Nursing, 35*(1), E7–E12.

Porath, C., & Pearson, C. (2013). The price of incivility. *Harvard Business Review, 91*(1–2), 114–121.

Princeton WordNet. Tendency. http://wordnetweb.princeton.edu/perl/webwn

Rogers, S. E., Thrasher, A. D., Miao, Y., Boscardin, W. J., & Smith, A. K. (2015). Discrimination in healthcare settings is associated with disability in older adults: Health and retirement study, 2008–2012. *Journal of General Internal Medicine, 30*(10), 1413–1420.

Ryan, R. M., & Deci, E. L. (2000). Self-determination theory and the facilitation of intrinsic motivation, social development, and well-being. *The American Psychologist, 55*(1), 68–78.

Shuck, B., Peyton Roberts, T., & Zigarmi, D. (2018). Employee perceptions of the work environment, motivational outlooks, and employee work intentions: An HR practitioner's dream or nightmare? *Advances in Developing Human Resources, 20*(2), 197–213.

Skinner, B. F. (1938). The Behavior of organisms: An experimental analysis, 1938. ISBN 1-58390-007-1, ISBN, 0-8741-487.x

Thesasurus.com. Uncivil. https://www.thesaurus.com/browse/uncivil

Tricco, A. C., Rios, P., Zarin, W., Cardoso, R., Diaz, S. Nincic, V., & Straus, S. E. (2018). Prevention and management of unprofessional behaviour among adults in the workplace: A scoping review. *PloS One, 13*(7), e0201187. doi:10.1371/journal.pone.0201187

U.S. News & World Report (2019). U.S. News Announces the 2019 Best Jobs. https://www.usnews .com/info/blogs/press-room/articles/2019-01-08/us-news-announces-the-2019-best-jobs

Vocabulary.com. Tendency. https://www.vocabulary.com/dictionary/tendency

Wiktionary.com. Tendency. https://en.wiktionary.org/wiki/tendency

Wiley, C. (1997). What motivates employees according to over 40 years of motivation surveys. *International Journal of Manpower, 18*(3), 263–280.

Williams, D. R., & Rucker, T. D. (2000). Understanding and addressing racial disparities in health care. *Health Care Financing Review, 21*(4), 75–90.

Windholz, G. (1997). Ivan P. Pavlov: An overview of his life and psychological work. *American Psychologist, 52*(9), 941–946. doi:10.1037/0003-066X.52.9.941

Winokur, S. (1971). Skinner's theory of behavior: An examination of BF Skinner's Contingencies of Reinforcement: A theoretical analysis 1. *Journal of the Experimental Analysis of Behavior, 15*(2), 253–259.

Worldometers. (June 11, 2020). Current World Population. https://www.worldometers.info/world -population/

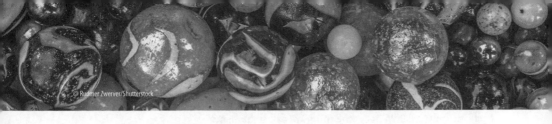
© Rudmer Zwerver/Shutterstock

CHAPTER 3

Sexualism: Reducing Sexual Harassment in Healthcare Workplaces

"No is a complete sentence."

– Anne Lamott, novelist and non-fiction writer

LEARNING OBJECTIVES

After completing this chapter, each reader will be able to:

- Define sexualism.
- Define sexual harassment.
- Compare and contrast behaviors that are considered sexual harassment, sexual assault, and rape. Analyze the thesis that various sexual behaviors by males toward females may have evolutionary roots.
- Describe and assess research that suggests the existence of linkages between "power" and sexual harassment across sex and gender, nations, and cultures.
- Outline implications of this research for strategies that can reduce power-related workplace sexual harassment.
- Analyze and critique the mechanisms by which humans behave in a way that is supportive of sexual harassment in the workplace.
- Apply the areas discussed in recommending strategies to increase workplace productivity by decreasing the prevalence and incidence of sexual harassment in the workplace.

▶ Introduction: Sexualism as the Framework for All Sexual Behaviors

The term **sexual harassment** refers to behaviors involving unwanted sexual attention. However, this chapter argues that the genesis of sexual harassment in healthcare workplaces is far more complex than is generally believed. More concretely, this chapter advances the concept that sexual harassment in workplaces is a result of the interaction of two other forces. These two other forces are 1) *sexualism*, a core human desire for sexual interaction among most humans; and 2) *propinquity*. Thus, first one must ask, "What is the thing we call sexualism?".

Sexualism

This term refers to a particular emphasis upon sex or sexuality in general according to the Merriam Webster dictionary. While some people view **sexualism** as referencing prejudice or discrimination, this is not actually true. The term literally refers to humanity's sexual desires, sexual interest, and sexual behaviors. However, all societies embrace behaviors that define the appropriate conditions under which sexual activities should be initiated and the terms under which they may be pursued. In general, workplaces are not considered an appropriate arena to pursue sexual interest.

The origins of cultural norms that define sexual behaviors are not new. Schulz (2005) suggests that even during the anthropological period in which hunting and gathering occurred in "workplaces" that consisted of forests and fields, cultural norms excluded these "workplaces" as settings appropriate for sexual behaviors. While anthropological research does not define the premise driving such expectations, such behaviors would have been a threat to the maximization of output. It is not surprising that in the far more complex environments that comprise contemporary workplaces, sexualism and/or sexually-related behaviors are actively discouraged based on written policies and procedures manuals.

For example, Robinson and Bennett (1995) introduced a framework to categorize the type of workplace behaviors that should not occur among workers. Categories identified and labeled as workplace deviant behaviors included theft, non-ethical acts, sexual harassment, and all output-reducing behaviors. Deviance was defined as any act that results in the performance of work-related activities at a level of quality significantly below the expected mean for the person's occupation. Property deviance refers to the use of items owned by the employer for non–work-related purposes. Political deviance describes the intrusion into the workplace of feelings, beliefs, and opinions regarding the distribution of power in ways that affect overall productivity. Finally, personal aggression of any kind against a co-worker was defined as forbidden. The use of the workplace for the pursuit of sexualistic purposes clearly falls into this latter category. Accordingly, workplaces have always been considered as inappropriate arenas for the expression of sexualism.

Despite such rules, workplaces have been used as contexts for the pursuit of both mutual and nonmutual sexual interests. Emery (2017), using data from a study by ReportLinker of 500 adults in the United States, found that 39% of people surveyed met through friends; 12% met in bars or at other social places; 9% met via sports, religion, or hobbies; 8% met using a dating app; and 15% met in the workplace. Leibowitz (2015), utilizing data collected through a Google Consumer Survey, discovered that for the 18–34 year olds interviewed, 39% met through friends, 22% met in another social setting, 9.4% met online, 5.8% met through a social setting, *and 17.9% met at work*. Such data suggest that despite the efforts of workplaces to eliminate the use of their premises for purposes associated with sexualisms, such behaviors occur and, in the process, may include sexual harassment or unwanted sexually-related behaviors. Yet, because of propinquity, sexualism has been around since precivilization and continues to exist in modern settings including workplaces.

▶ The Role of Propinquity in Transforming Sexualism into Sexual Harassment

The word, "**propinquity**" is derived from the Latin word for closeness or nearness, *propinquitas*. It defines the tendency of humans to create bonds with others based on physical proximity, feelings of kinship, affiliation, and/or other similarities.

Because early humans on the earth were limited to their geographic locations of residence due to an absence of worldwide travel, they lived in smaller societies around the world and were not able to easily meet other people. This resulted in propinquity existing within their societies. Humans create bonds with other human beings who are similar in geographical area, interests, basic needs, or other criteria. As cultures matured with newer technology and means of travel developed, propinquity continued to exist in neighborhoods, clubs, at cultural events, and not surprisingly, in places of employment. **BOX 3.1**. includes definitions for propinquity.

As the definitions of propinquity suggest, frequent interaction is the most basic element of propinquity (Pierce, Byrne, Aguinis, 1996, page 11). A now-classic article by Donald Marvin (1918) discusses "occupational propinquity" and its presence in all workplaces. The article discusses propinquity as it relates to choosing marriage partners in the late 19th century. Marvin maintains that the frequent and regular contact of women and men in the workplace caused "constant sexual stimulation" that ultimately influenced the choice of a marriage partner. Propinquity results in forming both nonsexual and sexual, interpersonal relationships. Propinquity and sexualism together directly led to the adoption of domains of single-sex education during earlier historical periods (Signorella, 2016). Single-sex workplaces were also once prevalent because of the assumption that the interaction of sexualism and propinquity would generate sexual harassment (Witz, 1990).

Stated differently, humans form and seek to become integrated into social groupings. In this regard, propinquity is regularly operative in peoples' lives including their home life, social life, education, and career or work life. For example, nonsexual or sexual bonds often form between roommates due to their proximity in the same environment from one day to the next. Festinger, Schachter, and

---

BOX 3.1 Definitions for Propinquity

- Propinquity—"nearness of blood" and/or "nearness in place or time." (Courtesy of Merriam Webster. Propinquity. https://www.merriam-webster.com/dictionary/propinquity).
- Propinquity (formal sense)—"the state of being close to someone or something; proximity" (technical sense); "close kinship." (Oxford Dictionary)

Back (1950), in a study of apartment dwellers, found that there was a connection between physical proximity and the development of interpersonal relationships of the people living on the same floor of the apartment building. John Gullahorn (1952) identified a positive correlation between physical proximity and the frequency of interactions among workers.

Moreover, businesses may unintentionally support propinquity in their hiring practices. In doing so, they may create an environment in which sexual harassment is likely to occur (Gautier, 2015). Specifically, workers are recruited based on certain qualifications that are needed for that particular industry. That is, the business that is hiring may seek prospective employees who will "fit" in the culture of the company and/or industry. Thus, co-workers who are hired and employed by the company will work in a culture that was attractive enough for them to accept the employment. Moreover, the hiring criterion will bring together persons who may share similar interests and/or other characteristics with other employees. It is these similarities coupled with physical proximity in the workplace on a regular basis that can lead to bonding. Many co-workers become friends and sustain interpersonal relationships while working in the same environment. But, the workplace can be an environment that inadvertently becomes a place where bonding based on sexual attraction may occur. But, it can also be an environment in which expressed sexual feelings are not reciprocated.

When a worker has sexual feelings for a coworker that are not reciprocated, the interested party may be rejected and will, as a result of the rejection, stop making advances. However, repeated advances may also occur. It is these types of scenarios that can result in sexual harassment in the workplace. While both males and females have been subjected to unwanted sexual overtures, Chatterjee (2018) reports that 81% of females have experienced unwanted sexually-related attention. Approximately 77% of females and 34% of males in this study had experienced verbal sexual harassment. Additionally, 51% of females and 17% of males had experienced unwelcome sexual touching. Approximately 38% of the women surveyed experienced harassment in the workplace. The accelerated interest in sexual harassment has led healthcare students and professionals to ask, "What is the magnitude and nature of sexual harassment in healthcare workplaces and how can such problems be remediated"? Before addressing this important question, sexual harassment needs to be defined from a legal perspective.

▶ Sexual Harassment as Defined by Title VII of the Civil Rights Act of 1964

Title VII of the Civil Rights Act of 1964 directly protects against any form of sex discrimination within work environments with 15 or more employees. Moreover, sexual harassment is considered to be a form of sex discrimination. Thus, the Equal Employment Opportunity Commission (EEOC) has defined sexual harassment as a behavior that violates Title VII of the Civil Rights Act of 1964. The standards indicated in **BOX 3.2** are used to support this interpretation.

As can be seen, sexual harassment is legally considered as a form of sexual discrimination. Yet, while it is true that sexual harassment is legally covered under laws that address sexual discrimination, this chapter argues that sexualism is actually a

---

BOX 3.2 EEOC's Definition of Sexual Harassment

"Unwelcome sexual advances, requests for sexual favors, or other verbal or physical conduct of a sexual nature constitute sexual harassment when this conduct explicitly or implicitly affects an individual's employment, unreasonably interferes with an individual's work performance, or creates an intimidating, hostile, or offensive work environment."

U.S. Equal Employment Opportunity Commission, Retrieved from https://www.eeoc.gov/eeoc/publications/fs-sex.cfm

---

different phenomenon than **sexism** in that the definition of the term sexualism is much broader. **BOX 3.3** examines some standardized definitions of sexism based on those that can be found in dictionaries.

In contrast, while some analysts have similarly defined sexualism, the term is much broader. **BOX 3.4** highlights these differences by introducing additional definitions to accompany those defined at the beginning of this chapter.

Sexualism, in its most basic forms, references sociobiological processes that relate to how the sexual systems in and between people are activated, the process by which relationships that can result in sexual interactions are best initiated, the relevance and appropriateness of workplaces for processes for sexual priming, and managing sexual stimuli within the norms of appropriate behavior that persist at any time. Stated differently, sexualisms reflect the sum of any individual's *human sexuality* and how it is expressed. Lehmiller in the book, *The Psychology of Human Sexuality* (2017), provides a comprehensive look at the complexities of human sexuality. Viewed from this perspective, sexualism, as it exists in workplaces, behaves differently from sexism but may be connected with sexism in generating the phenomena that we call sexual harassment. Because of the physical and social intimacy that workplaces embody on a day-to-day basis, the beginning, growth, and perpetuation of sexual harassment in workplaces can have adverse impacts on maximum productivity. Sexual harassment within the framework of sexism addresses this phenomenon.

BOX 3.3 Alternative Definitions of Sexism

- Sexism—Prejudice or discrimination based on sex (especially discrimination against women).
  (Courtesy of Merriam-Webster Dictionary. Sexism. https://www.merriam-webster.com/dictionary/sexism)
- Sexism—Actions based on a belief that particular jobs and activities are suitable only for women and others are suitable only for men.
  (Definition of 'Sexism' from Cambridge Dictionary, www.dictionary.cambridge.org, © Cambridge University Press. Used with permission.)

BOX 3.4 Definition of Sexualism

- Sexualism—Emphasis upon sex or sexuality as a major concern.
  (Courtesy of Merriam-Webster Dictionary. Sexualism. https://www.merriam-webster.com/dictionary/sexualism)

Sexual harassment is a workplace incivility that affects both males and females. All laws and policies regarding sex are crafted not only to protect "women" against sexual discrimination, but to also protect men. Sexual discrimination laws include actions that apply to all people whether their gender is biologically assigned or self-selected. The term, sexual harassment includes a number of behaviors including unwelcome sexual advances that occur within a work environment which are directed toward: 1) people seeking work; 2) an employee; 3) contractual workers; and/or, 4) clients or customers of an organization. Unwelcome sexual advances include behaviors such as those listed in **BOX 3.5**.

Sexualisms may include flirting. However, key characteristics differentiate sexual harassment and flirting. Specifically, sexualistic behaviors that mimic those listed below shift the behavior from flirting into the specific area that is legally defined as sexual harassment.

- Sexual attention that is unwanted comprises harassment for it then becomes offensive.
- Sexual attention that "disturbs and/or upsets" the recipient is harassment.
- Sexual attention that causes the recipient to feel threatened and/or intimidated is harassment.

Such behaviors create legal problems for both the individual and the healthcare institution that employs the harasser and the harassed. Additionally, these behaviors also reduce output maximization. Now-classic research by Crull (1982), DiTomaso (1989), and others have found that such experiences reduce motivation, self-confidence, and commitment to work. Xin et al. (2018), in a study of 210 workers in China, discovered that sexual harassment in the workplace actually generated a spillover effect that led to diminished quality in the marriages of workers. One theory is that this spillover effect may occur, in part, because the actual experiences of sexual harassment are further complicated by the absence of empathy for such experience within the workplace. McCord et al. (2018) completed a systematic review of literature that supports this perspective. These researchers discovered that when sexual harassment occurs in the workplace, general isolation occurs in males who do not perceive the behaviors as harassment. (These analysts also found that the collective research reveals that a parallel phenomenon occurs

---

BOX 3.5 Behaviors That Are Considered "Unwelcome Sexual Advances"

- Unwanted verbal remarks or discussions of sexual matters;
- Unwanted touching of any part of another person's body;
- Persistent and unwanted requests for a "date";
- Unnecessary and unwanted physical contact of any nature;
- Sexual motions;
- Unwanted jokes of a sexual nature;
- Exposing an individual to sexually explicit photos, videos, or other visible or audible materials;
- Making statements that have explicit, embedded, or even implied sexual innuendos; and
- Others.

by race/ethnicity.) The failure to find comfort among co-workers may, of course, create an even greater sense of alienation that spills over into other areas of the workers' life.

The impact of the harassment may affect the worker in another way that ultimately inhibits productivity. Wang et al. (2018), using sites in the United States and China, revealed that emphasizing productivity maximization is also diluted by an emphasis upon "...both major and minor revenge" (pg. 151).

Less output-inhibiting ways than "revenge" are also included in the responses to sexual harassment. Burgess et al. (2015), based on data collected from six different sites, found that sexual harassment is a standard part of the culture of assisted living institutions. Given its magnitude, this study found that rather than applying "revenge," workers used neutralizing behaviors such as non-engagement, redirection, and/or other strategies that allowed them to maintain the required levels of productivity.

In contrast, other workplaces have been far more adversely affected. Taylor, et al. (2017) identified a standard of support for sexual harassment in male majority occupations that was so extreme that it was considered the norm. The impact was so great that when sexual harassment was particularly aggressive, the victims of such behaviors required psychotherapy, pharmacotherapy and, in some cases, hospitalization. As a result, the impact on output maximization was greatly affected because the workers experienced lower levels of productivity. Because sexual harassment is also associated with turnover, transfer, and absenteeism (Merkin & Shah, 2014; Chan, Lam, Chow & Cheung, 2008; Laband & Lentz, 1998), sexual harassment can also adversely affect the victim's entire career. Additionally, the decreased productivity can increase costs and lower profits. Higher rates of employee turnover can also affect organizational effectiveness (Ton & Huckman, 2008; Staw, 1980). Thus, sexual harassment not only impacts the individual, it also affects the organization. Individuals who have experienced sexual harassment and/or **sexual assault** can develop long-standing and serious medical issues because as a person experiences sexual harassment or sexual assault, he or she is often traumatized. This trauma can lead to **somatization**.

Somatization occurs when the affected person internalizes his or her feelings and his or her body becomes ill. People who experience sexual harassment or sexual assault can suffer from mental illness and/or physical illness as a result (Thurston et al., 2018; Ho et al., 2010; Chan et al., 2008; Rospenda et al. (2005); Farley & Kaney, 1997; Lenhart, 1996). Some of the more common afflictions include stomach upset, Post-Traumatic Stress Disorder (PTSD), depression, thoughts of suicide, heart-related issues, sleep problems, high blood pressure, neck pain, and other symptoms or illnesses. Understandably, people who have experienced sexual harassment on the job tend to be absent from work more often. This can adversely affect their overall job quality, the overall capabilities of their employer's organization, and other life areas.

For example, Yang (2017), using data from more than 200,000 children and youth from more than 9,000 schools in 27 countries, determined that direct linkages exist between the existence of discrimination in general in the larger society and the pattern of truancy among children of immigrants. Stated differently, the losses that occur from sexual harassment and other forms of discrimination can adversely impact the society through a complex system of cause and effect.

It is important to remember that sexual harassment, sexual assault, and rape are different. Sexual harassment encompasses those actions that are of a sexual nature, i.e., catcalls, other inappropriate verbal speech, repeated sexual overtures, sexual advances, quid pro quo proposals, or other verbal or physical conduct of an unwelcome sexual nature. However, sexual assault refers to any behavior in which one individual touches another individual's body, including genitals, breasts, buttocks, lips, and/or other body parts for the purposes of sexual arousement and/or sexual pleasure without stated consent. Sexual assault may include rape. However, the various states in the country differentially define sexual assault as well as rape.

At one end of the spectrum, there are behaviors such as the exposure or viewing of another's buttocks, breasts, genitalia, etc. These actions represent sexual assault. Sexual assault is contact without permission with another individual's breasts, buttocks, or other body parts. Additionally, permission is needed for a person to take a photo of another. Since the advent of cell phone cameras, there have been reports of "upskirt" or "down blouse" photography wherein a male takes an unauthorized photo or video under the skirt or dress of a female, or of her bosom down her blouse, usually going undetected. In England and Wales, males in kilts have also been targeted with this type of action by females and are now protected by the law BBC (2018). Interestingly, America does not have laws specifically addressing this phenomenon. However, victims of such actions are protected through the Video Voyeurism Prevention Act of 2004.

Unwanted kisses are also defined as sexual assault. This is because any sexual activity without explicit consent is defined as sexual assault. However, sexual assault also references unwanted penetration whether by fingers, sexual organs, an object, etc. Moreover, in several states, sexual harassment and sexual assault mean the same thing although they have different meanings in other states. For example, in New Jersey, rape and sexual assault are now synonymous. Yet, in Pennsylvania, rape is based on the use of force to allow sexual access, while sexual assault is based on the absence of explicit consent. Thus, in Pennsylvania, rape sentences generally involve twice as much time in prison. In contrast, in Washington State, sexual assault is defined as rape as well as crimes with no sexual contact, but which were sexually motivated. This state-by-state differentiation allows juries to assign criminal sanctions to a greater range of sexual violations. These highly uncivil behaviors have been reported in all types of workplaces. Such behaviors are also considered "workplace injustice."

▶ Sexual Harassment in Healthcare Workplaces

Workplace injustice is defined as "discrimination, harassment, and bullying based on EEOC protected classes but also including sexual orientation, gender identity, health condition, and job title/position within the workplace" (Okechukwu, Souza, Davis & de Castro, 2014). Of particular concern to healthcare administrators, managers, and human resources managers, some evidence exists that this phenomenon exists in healthcare workplaces.

Jagsi (2018) asserts that "the problem of sexual harassment seems as severe in medicine as elsewhere, and standing up to harassers is hard for victims and institutions alike (pg. 209)." Bates et al. (2018) also suggest that behaviors that are defined as sexual harassment manifest themselves in healthcare workplaces at a level that parallels the magnitude of this phenomenon in entertainment and other industries. Specifically, people with greater power seek sexual access to unwilling partners and, in the process, create psychosocial damage. At the same time, the potential life "fallout" from reporting such circumstances includes penalties with lifelong consequences.

Kinard and Little (2002) begin their discussion by referencing a 1994 study of sexual harassments in hospitals—a set of healthcare institutions that employ the single largest number of healthcare workers. Gathering survey data over a 4.5 year time span, this 1994 study revealed a number of trends: 1) An accelerated increase in the number of formalized sexual harassment cases that were being filed in hospitals; and 2) A set of complaints in which more than 80% of all charges were for sexual advances that limited the maximization of output by creating a hostile environment. The second dominant form of sexual harassment was based on the effort of people in superior positions to negotiate sexual "favors" in exchange for workplace advancements (quid pro quo). "**Quid pro quo**" is a Latin term that translates to "something for something." One example of quid pro quo is **transactional sex** wherein sex is provided in direct exchange for a cash or non-cash payment.

Kinard and Little (2002) also indicate that sexual harassment in hospital environments has been characterized by growth. From 1994 to 1999, the number of Equal Employment Opportunity Commission (EEOC) cases filed against hospitals increased to almost 16,000. Moreover, sexual harassment charges were extensive. One large pharmaceutical company, Astra Pharmaceutical, literally paid almost $10 million ($9.95 million) as part of a sexual harassment claims case filed by the EEOC. Astra Pharmaceuticals is a worldwide company and is part of AstraZeneca. It employs between 5,001–10,000 workers according to its website at www.astrazeneca-us.com. The above cited sexual harassment case involved firing older female employees. They were replaced by single, younger female employees who, it was hoped, would be more responsive to sexual advances in the workplace.

The data for this case revealed that numerous formal complaints were lodged by nurses against coworkers of higher workplace rank. However, the perpetrators were not predominantly physicians. In fact, slightly less than 10% were physicians. The study did not clarify the specific positions held in hospital workplaces by these other 90% of perpetrators of sexual harassment. This case also demonstrates that contrary to sexism, sexual harassment also affects males. Several males also experienced this incivility. In fact, the EEOC reported that in 2017, 16.5% of all of their sexual harassment charges filed with the EEOC for sex-based harassment were filed by males (https://www.eeoc.gov/eeoc/statistics/enforcement/sexual_harassment_new.cfm).

Interestingly, males are harassed in the same way as females. The EEOC recognizes two illegal types of sexual harassment that can be filed with the agency. They handle "quid pro quo" (sexual coercion) and "hostile work environment" claims (https://www.eeoc.gov/laws/types/harassment.cfm). Any kind of behavior of a sexual or sexual innuendo nature that makes any employee (male or female) uncomfortable is known as a hostile work environment.

Sexual harassment in hospitals and other environments is a worldwide phenomenon. For example, sexual harassment is a major problem in India and other

South Asian countries. Sexual harassment has achieved such a magnitude that a newer term "**eve teasing**" has been coined for one particular type of sexual harassment that takes place mainly in public places (Talboys et al. 2017). This type of sexual harassment usually happens to strangers in public places and predominantly to young girls and women. A stranger may lightly touch, catcall, grope, or make sexual remarks to a passerby or passenger. However, sexual harassment in South Asia also exists in medical facilities. For example, Subedi et al. (2013) determined that 40.3% of a sample of 134 nurses from one public healthcare organization and three private nurses in Nepal had experienced sexual harassment at work. The forms of harassment that occurred most often were "hearing vulgar jokes, persons staring at their bodies, co-workers embracing them without their consent, and/or co-workers attempting to inappropriately touch them." Interestingly, such incidents were most frequent among nurses aged 20–29. Approximately 62.96% of the nurses who had experienced harassment were in this age group. Approximately 18.52% were aged 30–39, 14.8% were under age 20, and only 3.7% were over age 40. Thus, ageism interacted with sexualism to decrease sexual harassment among women over 40.

While unmarried women comprised 39.25% of nurses who had been sexually harassed, 40.75% of the women were married. Workplace harassment in Nepal was also a function of the nurses' body weight. Approximately 77.78% of the nurses in the sample who reported harassment had a body mass index (BMI) that fell between 18.5 and 29.9. In this particular study, 100% of the perpetrators were male. Approximately 37.03% of the harassers in this study were physicians, 25.93% were the patients' relatives, 18.52% were patients themselves, 11.11% were administrative staff including hospital administrators and managers, and 7.4% were technical staff.

There is evidence that more sexual harassment incidents occur in hospitals than in other healthcare organizations. Rege (2017), using EEOC data obtained from BuzzFeed News, identified 170,000 sexual harassment claims that were filed with the EEOC over the 21-year period from 1995 to 2016. This represents a mean of 8,095.24 cases per year. These data are important because they provide a loosely defined portrait of the distributional pattern of sexual harassment across different healthcare workplaces. This article states that general medical and surgical hospitals had 3,085 claims. Thus, they appear to have the most cases of sexual harassment. This is not surprising given that hospitals employ a larger proportion of the overall healthcare workforce. Ambulatory healthcare service facilities ranked second with 1,911 cases, and nursing care facilities were third with 1,530 complaints. However, 50 or more cases were also filed by workers in medical laboratories (436), physician offices (382), home healthcare services (314), direct health and medical insurance carriers (254), offices of other miscellaneous healthcare practitioners (140), specialty hospitals (81), psychiatric and substance abuse hospitals (73), ambulance services (51), and other outpatient care centers (50). It becomes particularly important to examine research on sexual harassment as a threat to output maximization in healthcare workplaces.

But, healthcare workplaces do not lead the nation in terms of sexual harassment. In an analysis of EEOC data, Frye (2017) found that from 2005–2015, health care and social assistance ranked fourth in the number of sexual harassment cases that were filed. The accommodation and food services industry ranked first with 14.23%

of all cases. Retail trade was second with 13.44%, manufacturing "housed" 11.72% of all cases, and health care and social assistance tied for third place with 11.48% of all cases. Hospitals, as the largest healthcare workplace, have had a number of high profile legal cases. Evans (2018) reports on a $168 million settlement in a 2014 sexual harassment suit brought against Catholic Healthcare West. Other cases could also be cited.

Sexual harassment also occurs with patients and/or patients' families and not only with other employees. Friborg et al. (2017), in a study of 7,603 employees and supervisors from five different occupations in healthcare in Denmark, researched whether the depressive symptoms associated with workplace sexual harassment were more severe when harassment occurred by other workers or by clients. This study revealed that employees harassed by other employees were more depressed than those harassed by clients, patients, customers, etc. The results are not surprising considering that the "dosage" of sexual harassment is higher and more continuous with colleagues than with customers/clients/patients. Moreover, a higher depression rate among employees subjected to harassment by other employees may stem from the fact that workers spend more time at their workplaces than anywhere else. This increases the odds of a greater frequency of such behaviors. While wishing to stay employed, the employee continues working. Yet, because they dread their daily experiences, they sometimes develop depressive symptoms.

Sexual Harassment in Non-Hospital Healthcare Workplaces

The focus so far has primarily been on sexual harassment in hospitals. This phenomenon also manifests in other healthcare workplaces. In a survey of sexual harassment, sexual aggression, and workplace aggression and violence among 1,214 homecare workers in the State of Oregon, Hanson et al. (2018) found that approximately 38.5% of workers had experienced sexual harassment or sexual aggression. In many cases, these behaviors were accompanied by verbal aggression and/or actual workplace violence (23.6%). As in other workplaces, such behaviors resulted in obstacles to output maximization due to increased stress, depression, overall burnout, and difficulty sleeping.

Emergency medicine, as a unique area of hospitals, also experienced very high levels of sexual harassment. Schnapp et al. (2016) reported that 52% or 62 of 119 emergency medicine residents serving patients in hospitals in New York had experienced sexual harassment. Moreover, 66% literally experienced one or more acts of physical violence. Emergency room patients have also reported experiencing sexual harassment or more grievous actions by their medical handlers. For example, the New York Times (2017) reported that a New York court handed down a 2-year sentence to a doctor in response to the severity of his sexual actions against an emergency room patient. (Other women had also complained to the medical facility regarding this physician's sexual harassment toward them.) Similarly, Burgess et al. (2018) completed a study of sexual harassment experienced by workers in six assisted living facilities. Multiple occurrences of sexual harassment also occurred in these environments.

Current Research Regarding the Causes of Sexual Harassment in Healthcare and Other Workplaces

A number of observations and theories have materialized regarding the causes of sexual harassment in health and nonhealth workplaces. Wood (2018), for example, argued that, "workplace flirtations and romance are a reality, but it may be difficult for some to recognize when the line between welcome flirtations and unwelcome harassment has been crossed." For the purposes of this discussion, this phenomenon has been labeled the "Misread Courting Signals Hypothesis." In order to explain this hypothesis, one must first review what attraction signals look like and how they have been previously sent, received, and interpreted.

Lindgren et al. (2008) conducted a literature review of studies that have shown that perceptual differences between males and females and/or same sex individuals may be involved in sexual harassment behavior. These authors explained the chain of events that may occur in several different ways. **BOX 3.6** lists some of these sources of miscommunication.

While the described hypothesis may help to understand one type of sexual harassment, this concept does not explain quid pro quo harassment. In some respects, sexual harassment in hospital work environments can be partially attributed to miscommunication regarding sexual attraction and the overly aggressive pursuit

---

BOX 3.6   The Misread/Courting/Signals/Hypothesis

- Premise #1: Sexual behavior is critical to the continuation of humankind.
- Premise #2: Sexual attraction is prerequisite to mutually agreed upon sexual interactions in psychosocially healthy individuals.
- Premise #3: The terms of sexual interaction may differ between humans by sex, culture, and other factors.
- Premise #4: Therefore, individuals are required to communicate several types of information such as: a) Is there sexual attraction? b) If so, is there a high probability of a sexual interaction? c) If so, what will be the terms of the sexual interaction?
- Except in the case of sex workers, the key questions listed above cannot be answered through direct question-and-answer communications in most of the world's cultures because to do so would be considered an incivility.
- As a result, the terms of mutually consensual sex are shifted from the realm of the contractual as was true in historical periods when marriages were arranged, to the nebulous realm of social signals.
- The use of these signals is, according to a number of researchers, differentially translated by males and females. If such signals were more directly expressed and responded to by the two people involved, some degree of sexual harassment would not occur.
- Other research indicates that people in the workplace and beyond understand the role of biological "signals" in sexual attraction. Gregoire (2015) also summarizes research from several studies that concluded that males and females also send biological "signals" to each other that support sexual attraction.
- Understanding such elements may also support more rational sexual behavior in and out of the workplace.

of sexual opportunity. In contrast, quid pro quo harassment explicitly acknowledges that an imbalanced sexual attraction exists. An effort is made to substitute actual or potential economic or other gain in an effort to negotiate sexual access. Accordingly, interpersonal outreach goes from one that is inclusive of romance-plus-sex, to one that is based on sex as a business.

This process differs significantly from attraction-only based sex. Karandashev and Fata (2014) completed an analysis of attraction in 29 females and 17 males aged 18–38 who varied by race/ethnicity. These individuals found that attraction emerged as the sum of behavioral, physiological, cognitive, and emotional aspects of the interaction. Attraction is defined by the authors based on other researchers, as "... an empowering emotion and a positive attitude of one person to another, displayed by the desire to approach and be closer to another person" (Newcomb 1961). Thus, sexual attraction is emotionally and physically based. However, while physical attraction may include sexual attraction, it is much broader because it may not be accompanied by the desire for sexual intimacy. When quid pro quo harassment occurs in the workplace, one person desires sexual intimacy while the other does not. Accordingly, social and/or financial capital gains supplement the absence of sexual attraction by the uninterested person. Nurse Leader Insider (2018) cites recent cases of quid pro quo as well as hostile workplace harassment that have occurred in the recent past in healthcare workplaces.

▶ Solutions to Sexual Harassment in Healthcare and Other Workplaces

Employers seek to prevent sexual harassment. Two main strategies that are used include: 1) Didactic workplace *training courses*; and 2) Having clear and user-friendly *processes* for reporting and responding to sexual harassment when it occurs in the workplace. A recent online article by Julia Belluz (November 14, 2017) calculated the value of the anti-harassment training industry in the United States as having reached approximately One Billion Dollars! The size of the sexual harassment training industry is projected to grow even more since legislators across party lines are advocating for mandatory anti-sexual harassment training in 90% of workplaces.

While such a policy initially generates enthusiasm, further reflection causes hesitancy. This is because no current research exists to suggest that didactic training programs on sexual harassment are effective! Moreover, some analysts would argue that the purpose of training on sexual harassment was not designed as a workplace prevention practice. Some analysts argue that the sexual harassment courses were designed as a protection against litigation! However, the argument also supports the idea that the ineffectiveness of sexual harassment training can be located in limitations in the general public health response to healthcare crises. Educating the public regarding the nature of the health issue is a primary approach that is often used. Specifically, the current models of intervention used begin with education about the public health issue. But health education alone is insufficient. Although education improves understanding of healthcare problems, health education does not directly and linearly lead to behavioral change. Rather, fundamental changes are needed in the structure of our society at the **macro-** and **micro-levels**.

In order to address quid pro quo harassment, the operation of power must be analyzed. Sexual harassment commonly embodies an imbalanced distribution of power. There are many accounts of situations in which a supervisor or other senior worker harasses a lower-ranked worker. This suggests that several solutions can be applied to the problem of the power imbalance in the workplace as a source of workplace sexual harassment. First, healthcare workplaces must ensure that the distribution of power doesn't reproduce itself by excluding key subgroups. This result is achieved through statistics. Second, every work environment must include an easy-to-use online platform for the reporting of sexual harassment. Third, every organization may wish to analyze data on those applicants who were selected for positions of power in order to ensure that systematic practices are not manipulating hiring and promotion outcomes toward some subgroups over others. This discussion implies that each organization may best serve itself by utilizing methods of appraisal and selection that generate the closest thing to a normal curve. Fourth, the criteria used for hiring may involve completing a comprehensive background check on all candidates for "powerful" positions in each organization. These background checks are needed because, according to psychologists, the most powerful predictor of the future is what occurred in the past.

Additionally, the human resources department may wish to introduce a policy that involves using an ethics tool as part of the screening process. There are a number of valid and reliable ethics instruments. For example, the ARECCI Ethics Screening Tool (Hagen et al., 2007), the PHO Risk Screening Tool (Ondrusek et al., 2015), the Clinical Ethics Screening Tool (Labrador-Grenfell Health, 2005), and/ or others can be used. While applicants and/or employees may positively position themselves and create a good perception, valuable information can still be obtained. Conducting a background check indicates to each candidate that the organization is committed to an ethical workplace.

In order to minimize imbalanced power as a tool to support sexual harassment, employers may wish to hold group and individual sessions led by a trained therapist as part of an orientation process for higher-level staff. These sessions will help to bring about ethical change. This may prevent people from abusing their power. However, the purpose of the sessions is not to increase the employees' knowledge of sexual harassment laws. Rather, the sessions would be group therapy sessions designed to prevent or reduce the abuse of power.

Indeed, evidence exists that all people in positions of power need to undergo therapy as a preventive measure to the abuse of power. Robust research in the area of behavioral health confirms that there are direct linkages between power and the abuse of power. In a 2013 article, "The Essential Tension Between Leadership and Power," Maner and Case cite some of this research. In a 2003 article entitled From Power to Action, researchers Galinsky, Gruenfeld, and Magee argue that independent of whether power is held by males, females, Caucasians, or others, the aged or the young, LGBTQ individuals and/or any other groups, certain common behavioral patterns occur. One of these is a process that is called "**disinhibition**," a psychological process in which persons rid themselves of social/ethical restraints.

Accordingly, if behavioral and mental health therapy is provided when the employee first assumes the position of increased power, it may ultimately prevent this behavior. Other research also support this argument. An article by Gruenfeld et al. (2008) suggested that power itself can cause individuals to not view others humanistically. Rather, it generates an unannounced, unconscious perspective that prompts them to see others as "objects" and not as human "subjects" with feelings. This process is called *objectification*. Objectification, as it relates to sexual harassment, is the treatment of the other person as an object and not necessarily as a whole person. The harasser sees the other person as being without thought or feeling and merely as an object capable of satisfying the harasser's personal needs. Basically, the harassed person is viewed as a tool and not as a person. The harassed becomes an object of sexual desire. Slabu and Guinote (2010) argue that there may exist an instinctive response that prompts an individual to use how much and/or how little power he or she has while trying to satisfy his or her own needs and objectives. Stated differently, as any individual obtains more power, his or her own instinct is to use this power to serve his or her own needs. Accordingly, preventive behavior therapy is necessary as individuals' power grows so that these processes can be consciously contained. Again, this leads to the conclusion that preventive therapy is needed from the very moment power is bestowed to help individuals preempt these behavioral changes.

These processes fully explain sexual harassment in the workplace that occurs between people in positions of power and those who have less power. In fact, Kuntsman and Maner (2011), another group of researchers cited in Maner and Case's (2013) article, believe that the pursuit of "objects" to satisfy sexual desires increases as power grows. Thus, the need for preventive therapy is crucial. However, another type of training must also accompany the use of preventive therapy.

Those who have less power and who are at greater risk of becoming "objects" in the lives of those with power require a unique type of "Empowerment Training" that teaches them why they should not allow the other person to "oppress" them (Collier, 1977). For workplace sexual harassment to flourish, a system of sanctions must exist that "rewards" the harassed for remaining silent and that "punishes" the harassed for speaking up. This is often true because the person who is harassed may have families to support and other needs that demand income and career paths. Therefore, unique strategies may be required to support those who are or have been harassed. First, Empowerment Training may be needed that not merely describes processes for reporting incidents of sexual harassment. Rather, this training must also provide the behavioral health support needed to assist the harassed person in overcoming the fear of the sanctions that generate silence. The harassed are also in need of the behavioral health support services from sources within or external to the workplace.

As mentioned previously, "oppressive" relationships are sustained in a society through a system of sanctions that include rewards for cooperating with "oppression" and punishment for refusing to "cooperate." This system regulates behavior so effectively that these responses become automated and/or habitual. Chi (2016) reports on research by Nicole Calakos et al. This study revealed that when behavior becomes a habit in mice, the "stop" and "go" behaviors in the brain literally begin to function differently. Specifically, the "go" and "stop" signals reverse themselves. These findings can be applied to sexual harassment dynamics. The person of lesser power may become so accustomed to incivilities that their brains literally become "wired" to sustain previously learned behaviors. Because of this process, the intensity of the training needed to empower these individuals will be quite high. It is not clear whether empowerment training will be fully effective. Yet, empowerment seminars and training can at least help the harassed to understand that: 1) there is a need for changes in their responses; 2) systems and processes are in place to ensure that their "speaking out" will result in organizational action; 3) they will not be "punished" for speaking up; and 4) even if they experience negative consequences, they have chosen to become a component in a process of change. Again, the idea that treatment is needed by both "power abusers" and "power-abused persons" is an important premise. Yet, instead of using behavioral health interventions, in the past, workplaces have offered brief, in-person or online sexual harassment training rather than behavioral and mental health prevention therapy. It is less than surprising that these methods have proven ineffective.

Sometimes sexual harassment occurs between two people in the workplace who are equally powerful. However, while power-based sexual harassment requires one type of preventive strategy, sexual harassment that begins with flirtation requires something different since flirting in the workplace can transform into sexual harassment. Although employees have received sexual harassment training, it does not allow employees to understand the dynamics of flirting. Thus, training may be needed that is called, "The Language of Flirting."

Gersick and Kurzban (2014) describe flirting as "…a class of courtship signaling that conveys the signalers' intentions and desirability to the intended while minimizing the costs that would accompany an overt courtship attempt." Stated differently, while flirting behavior occurs between all animal species to signal sexual interest, the processes of sending and interpreting romantic and/or sexual interest among humans is far more subtle and, as a result, can be misinterpreted. This suggests that in some cases, the source of sexual harassment in the workplace may occur as a result of signal misinterpretation. Hall, Xing, and Brooks (2014) analyzed data from 52 male/female pairs. Their study found that it was easier for participants to define flirting absence rather than its presence. An individual can easily misread the actions of another person. Interestingly, in a second study, one of these researchers also discovered that female flirting was more accurately interpreted than male flirting. However, some researchers have found that males often mistake female friendliness as flirting.

An array of research has identified signals of "flirting" between two people and the places that are considered "flirting appropriate." Flirting is social body language. Prolonged eye contact, slight touches, giggling and playfulness, leaning "in"—all of these behaviors denote flirtation. Appropriate settings for flirting include: parties, celebrations, night clubs, college campuses, weddings and religious events, and other social events. But, flirting in the workplace may be directly viewed as a form of sexual harassment and is considered as an inappropriate workplace behavior. A number of factors support this conclusion. In the past, flirting in selected areas of work environments was considered acceptable. These areas included cafeterias, coffee areas, office parties, etc. However, the seriousness of the need to avoid hostile work environments suggests that the emotions associated with dating and mating threatens the workplace. Thus, each organization must develop its own guidelines for flirting and dating in the workplace. For example, such preventive guidelines may inhibit the sending of texts and emails that could be considered inappropriate. Moreover, the guidelines should be included in the Employees' Handbook and the Employees' Manual. These documents should be distributed to all employees, contractors, vendors, and others who frequent the workplace. Accordingly, there are certain behaviors that employees should avoid if they are in a "no flirting" work environment. One example is prolonged eye contact. That is often interpreted as flirting. Prolonged eye contact is generally considered flirting if it involves silently gazing into another person's eyes for more than a second or two. (However, if one is discussing work, eye contact is considered a sign of attentiveness.) But eye contact that travels over an individual's body parts during conversations is not considered flirting. It is considered sexual aggression.

Invading someone's personal space is also problematic. Edward T. Hall (1963), an American anthropologist, introduced the term "proxemics" to describe the science of personal space. He defined physical zones for the physical closeness of one human to another. The furthest zone is the public distance zone, which is approximately 12 feet. A person whom the other person does not know nor has ever met (i.e., the public at large) is in this group. The second zone is for people who are casually known through social channels but not considered "friends." The third space (a length of 2–5 feet) is for personal friends and family. This zone is for people whom we know and trust. Finally, the closest zone is that of intimacy and is for those people with whom the person has an intimate connection or relationship. Considering these personal space guidelines, being closer than 3–5 feet away from someone in the workplace can be viewed as an invasion of personal space. Standing 1'6" or less from a person is a form of sexual harassment because that space is usually considered an area reserved for those with a very, very intimate relationship. However, there may be times in a workplace where there are crowded hallways or tight spaces that a worker has to navigate in the course of the workday.

One problem that complicates charges of sexual harassment is misinterpretation. Often, individuals cannot appropriately "read" the other person's body language. However, researchers have identified signs of discomfort based on body language. Researchers label this as "nonverbal leakage." Such behaviors may include tenseness, arms folded very tightly, moving away, the absolute absence of eye contact, or the absence of animation. This nonverbal leakage may signal that the other person is very uncomfortable. However, other behaviors definitely signal flirting. These include:

- Touch is considered flirting even if it is a slight arm touch;
- Vocal signals can suggest flirtation;
- Unsolicited disclosure of personal information can be considered flirting;
- Playful teasing can be interpreted as a form of flirtation; and
- Other.

Efforts should be taken to minimize flirtation in the workplace. However, it is important to understand that if a workplace romance does emerge, if one party wishes to break it off and the other party doesn't, it does become a form of sexual harassment. Other types of sexual harassment other than flirting include: 1) unsolicited sexual teasing; 2) jokes (vulgar, etc.); 3) off-color remarks; and 4) personal questions.

▶ Summary

In some respects, healthcare workplaces embody many of the characteristics that are supportive of the gestation and growth of sexual harassment. Tecco et al. (2018) cite data that reveal several gender disparities in power relationships within healthcare workplaces from hospitals to digital health entities. This power imbalance further propagates sexual harassment given the over-representation of females in the overall healthcare industry. However, the dynamics of sexual harassment in healthcare and other environments are far more complex than is commonly understood. This chapter has generated additional research, discussion, and solutions to this unique aspect of sexualism so that progress toward output maximization can be accelerated.

Wrap-Up

Review Questions

1. The chapter argues that sexualism, when combined with propinquity, can generate sexual harassment in healthcare and other workplaces. Conduct research that allows you to support or reject such an argument.
2. How many types of sexual harassment in healthcare workplaces were discussed in this chapter? How do the proposed solutions in this chapter differ?
3. Based on your research on human resources law, can a healthcare workplace legally mandate therapy for people who supervise other healthcare workers?

Key Terms and Concepts

Disinhibition
Eve teasing
Macro-level
Micro-level
Propinquity
Quid pro quo

Sexism
Sexual assault
Sexual harassment
Sexualism
Somatization
Transactional Sex

References

Bates, C. K., Jagsi, R., Gordon, L. K., Travis, E., Chatterjee, A., Gillis, M., Means, O., Chaudron, L., Ganetzky, R., Gulati, M., Fivush, B., Sharma, P., Grover, A., Lautenberger, D., & Flotte, T. (2018). It is time for zero tolerance for sexual harassment in academic medicine. *Academic Medicine, 93*(2), 163–165.

Belluz, J. (2017). Congress is making harassment trainings mandatory. Science shows they don't work. Retrieved from https://www.vox.com/science-and-health/2017/10/24/16498674/corporate -harassment-trainings-dont-work

British Broadcasting Corporation (BBC). (2018). Upskirting ban 'also protects men in kilts.' https:// www.bbc.com/news/uk-politics-44542051

Britannica Dictionary. Sexism. https://www.britannica.com/topic/sexism

Burgess, E. O., Barmon, C., Moorhead, J. R., Perkins, M. M., & Bender, A. A. (2018). That is so common everyday…everywhere you go! Sexual harassment of workers in assisted living. *Journal of Applied Gerontology, 37*(4), 397–418. doi:10.1177/0733464816630635

Cambridge Dictionary. Sexism. https://dictionary.cambridge.org/us/dictionary/english/sexism

Chan, K-S., Lam, C. B., Chow, S. Y., & Cheung, S. F. Examining the job-related, psychological, and physical outcomes of workplace sexual harassment: A meta-analytic review. *Psychology of Women Quarterly, 32*(4), 362. doi:10.1111/j.1471-6402.2008.00451.x

Chatterjee, R. (2018). A new survey finds 81 percent of women have experienced sexual harassment, *NPR,* https://www.npr.org/sections/thetwo-way/2018/02/21/587671849/a-new-survey-finds -eighty-percent-of-women-have-experienced-sexual-harassment

Chi, K. R. (2016). Why are habits so hard to break? *Duke Today,* in Campus, Medicine, Research. https://today.duke.edu/2016/01/habits

Collier, B. J. (1977). Economics, psychology and racism: A model of oppression. *Journal of Black Psychology, 3*(3), 50–60.

Collins Dictionary. Sexualism. https://www.collinsdictionary.com/us/dictionary/english/sexualism

Crull, P. (1982). Stress effects of sexual harassment on the job: implications for counseling. *American Journal of Orthopsychiatry, 52*(3), 539–544.

Dictionary.com. Sexism. https://www.dictionary.com/browse/sexism

DiTomaso, N. (1989). Sexuality and the workplace: discrimination and harassment. In J. Hearn, D. L. Sheppard, P. Tancred-Sheriff, & G. Burrell (Eds.), *The Sexuality of Organization*, (pp. 71–90). Sage Publications, London.

EEOC. Title VII of the Civil Rights Act of 1964. https://www.eeoc.gov/laws/statutes/titlevii.cfm

EEOC Sexual Harassment. EEOC https://www.eeoc.gov/eeoc/publications/fs-sex.cfm

EEOC Sex-based harassment. Charges Alleging Sex-Based Harassment (Charges filed with EEOC) FY 2010–FY 2018 https://www.eeoc.gov/eeoc/statistics/enforcement/sexual_harassment_new.cfm

EEOC. Harassment. https://www.eeoc.gov/laws/types/harassment.cfm

Emery, L. R. (2017). Where people are actually meeting their partners today, Bustle, https://www.bustle.com/p/where-people-are-actually-meeting-their-partners.

Evans, G. (2018). #MeToo in medicine? Sexual harassment in healthcare, *RELIAS Media* (Formerly AHC Media), https://www.reliasmedia.com/articles/142185-metoo-in-medicine-sexual-harassment-in-healthcare

Farley, M., & Keaney, J. C. (1997). Physical symptoms, somatization, and dissociation in women survivors of childhood sexual assault. *Womens Health, 25*(33), 33–45.

Festinger, L., Schachter, S., & Back, K. (1950). The spatial ecology of group formation. In L. Festinger, S. Schachter, & K. Back (Eds.), *Social pressure in informal groups*, 1950. Chapter 4.

Friborg, M. K., Hansen, J. V., Aldrich, P. T., Folker, A. P., Kjaer, S., Nielsen, M. B., … Madsen, I. E. H. (2017). Workplace sexual harassment and depressive symptoms: A cross-sectional multilevel analysis comparing harassment from clients or customers to harassment for other employees amongst 7603 Danish employees from 1041 organizations. *BMC Public Health, 17*(1), 675.

Frye, J. (2017). Not Just the Rich and Famous; Washington, D.C.: Center for American Progress, Washington D.C. https://www.americanprogress.org

Galinsky, A. D., Gruenfeld, D. H., & Magee, J. C. (2008). From power to action. *Journal of Personality and Social Psychology, 85*(3), 453–466.

Gautier, C. (2015). The psychology of work: Insights into successful working practices, Kogan Page Publishers.

Gersick, A., & Kurzban, R. (2014). Covert sexual signaling: Human flirtation and implications for other social species. *Evolutionary Psychology, 12*(3), 549–569. doi:10.1177/14747049140200305

Gregoire, C. (2015). The strange science of sexual attraction. *Science*, https://www.huffingtonpost.com/2015/02/14/science-of-attraction-_n_6661522.html

Gruenfeld, D. H., Inesi, M. E., Magee, J. C., & Galinsky, A. D. (2008). Power and the objectification of social targets. *Journal of Personality and Social Psychology, 95*(1), 111–127. doi:10.1037/0022-3514.95.1.111

Gullahorn, J. T. (1952). Distance and friendship as factors in the gross interaction matrix. *Sociometry, 15*(1–2), 123–134.

Hagen, B., O'Beirne, M., Desai, S., Stingl, M., Pachnowski, C. A., & Hayward, S. (2007). Innovations in the ethical review of health-related quality improvement and research: The Alberta Research Ethics Community Consensus Initiative (ARECCI). *Healthcare Policy, 2*(4), e164.

Hall, E. T. (1963). A system for the notation of proxemic behavior. *American Anthropologist, 65*, 1003–1026.

Hall J. A., Xing C., & Brooks S. (2014). Accurately detecting flirting. Error management theory, the traditional sexual script, and flirting base rate. doi:10.1177/0093650214534972

Hanson, G. C., Perrin, N. A., Moss, H., Lahainer, N., & Glass, N. (2015). Workplace violence against homecare workers and its relationship with workers health outcomes: A cross-sectional study. *BMC Public Health, 15*(11). doi:10.1186/s12889-014-1340-7

Ho, I. K., Dinh, K. T., Bellefontaine, S. A., & Irving, A. L. Sexual harassment and posttraumatic stress symptoms among Asian and white women. (2012) *Journal of Aggression, Maltreatment & Trauma, 21*(1), 95–113. doi:10.1080/10926771.2012.633238

Jagsi, R. (2018). Sexual harassment in medicine - #MeToo, *The New England Journal of Medicine, 378*(3), 209–211. doi:10.1056/NEJM, 1715962

Karandashev, V., & Fata, B. (2014). Change in physical attraction in early romantic relationships. *Interpersona: An International Journal on Personal Relationships, 8*(2), doi:10.5964/ojpr.v8.2.167

Kinard, J., & Little, B. (2002). Sexual harassment in the healthcare industry: A follow-up inquiry, *The Health Care Manager, 20*(4), 46–52.

Kunstman, J. W., & Maner, J. K. (2011). Sexual overperception: Power, mating motives, and biases in social judgment. *Journal of Personality and Social Psychology, 100*(2), 282–294. doi:10.1037/a0021135.

Labrador-Grenfell Health (2005). Clinical Ethics Screening Tool. Retrieved https://www.lghealth.ca/your-health/programs-and-services/ethics-service/

Laband, D. N., & Lentz, B. F. (1998). The effects of sexual harassment on job satisfaction, earnings, and turnover among female lawyers. *Industrial and Labor Relations Review, 51*(4). doi:10.1177/001979399805100403

Lehmiller, J. J. (2017). *The psychology of human sexuality*, 2nd Ed. John Wiley & Sons, Ltd. Southern Gate, Chichester, West Sussex, PO19 85Q UK.

Lenhart, S. (1996). Physical and mental health aspects of sexual harassment. In D. K. Shrier (Ed.), *Clinical practice series, No. 38. Sexual harassment in the workplace and academia: Psychiatric Issues,* 21–38. Arlington, VA, US: American Psychiatric Association.

Leibowitz, L. (2015). The way most people meet their significant others is probably not what you think, *MIC,* https://mic.com/articles/112062/the-way-most-people-meet-their-significant-others-is-not-what-you-think#.7BvB2t9Ta

Lindgren, K. P., Parkhill, M. R., George, W. H., & Hendershot, C. S. (2008). Gender differences in perceptions of sexual intent: A qualitative review and integration. *Psychology of Women Quarterly, 32*(4), 423–439. doi:10.1111/j.1471-6402 2008.00456.X

MacMillan Dictionary. Propinquity. https://www.macmillandictionary.com/us/dictionary/american/propinquity

Maner J. K., & Case, C. R. (2013). The essential tension between leadership and power: Why power corrupts – and how to prevent it. *Psychological Science Agenda,* Science Brief. October 2013. http://www.apa.org/science/about/psa/2013/10/leadership-power.aspx

Marvin, D. M. (1918). Occupational propinquity as a factor in marriage selection. *Publications of the American Statistical Association, 16*(123), 131–150.

McCord, M. A., Joseph, D. L., Dhanani, L. Y., & Beus, J. M. (2018). A meta-analysis of sex and race differences in perceived workplace misstatement. *Journal of Applied Psychology, 103*(2), 137–163. doi:10/1057/apl0000250

Merkin, R. S., & Shaw, M. K. (2014). The impact of sexual harassment on job satisfaction, turnover intentions, and absenteeism: Findings from Pakistan compared to the United States. *Springerplus, 3,* 215. doi:10.1186/2193-1801-3-215

Merriam Webster. Sexualism. https://www.merriam-webster.com/dictionary/sexualism

Merriam Webster. Propinquity. https://www.merriam-webster.com/dictionary/propinquity

Merriam Webster Sexism. https://www.merriam-webster.com/dictionary/sexism

New Dictionary of Cultural Literacy 3rd Edition, (2002). Sexism. Houghton Mifflin Harcourt Publishing Company. Boston | New York.

New York Times. January 23, 2017. Manhattan doctor is sentenced to 2 years in prison for sexually abusing patients. https://www.nytimes.com/2017/01/23/nyregion/manhattan-doctor-david-newman-prison-sexual-abuse.html

Newcomb, T. M. (1961). The acquaintance process. New York: Holt, Rinehart, and Winston.

Nurse Leader Insider. (March 8, 2018). Not Tolerated: Sexual Harassment in Healthcare, www.hcpro.com/WRS-330941-868/NOT-Tolerated

Okechukwu, C. A., Souza, K., Davis, K. D., & de Castro, A. B. (2014). Discrimination, harassment, abuse, and bullying in the workplace: Contribution of workplace injustice to occupational health disparities. *American Journal of Industrial Medicine, 57*(5), 573–586. doi:10.1002/ajim.22221

Ondrusek, N. K., Willison, D. J., Haroun, V., Bell, J. A., & Bornbaum, C. C. (2015). A risk screening tool for ethical appraisal of evidence-generating initiatives. *BMC Medical Ethics, 16*(1), 47.

Oxford Dictionary. Propinquity. https://www.lexico.com/en/definition/propinquity

Oxford Dictionary. Sexualism. https://www.lexico.com/en/definition/sexualism

Pierce, C. A., Byrne, D., & Aguinis, H. (1996). Attraction in organizations: A model of workplace romance. *Journal of Organizational Behavior, 17*(1), 5-32.

Rege, A. (2017). Report: At least 3,085 hospital employees filed sexual harassment claims between 1995 and 2016. Becker's Hospital Review.

Robinson, S. L., & Bennett, R. J. (1995). A typology of deviant workplace behaviors: A multidimensional scaling study. *Academy of Management Journal, 38*(2), 555–572. doi:10.5465/256693

Rospenda, K. M., Richman, J. A., Ehmke, J. L. Z., & Zlatoper, K. W. (2005). Is workplace harassment hazardous to your health? *Journal of Business and Psychology, 20*. doi:10.1007/s10869-005 -6992-y

Schnapp, B. H., Slovis, B. H., Shah, A. D., Fant, A. L., Gisondi, M. A., Shah, K. H., & Lech, C. A. (2016). Workplace violence and harassment against emergency medicine residents. *Western Journal of Emergency Medicine, 17*(5), 567–573. doi:10.5811/westjem.2016.630446

Schulz, M. (2005). Sex in the stone age pornography in clay: Part II: How promiscuous were prehistoric humans? *Spiegel Online*, http://www.spiegel.de/international/spiegel/sex-in-the -stone-age-pornography-in-clay-a-350042-2.html

Signorella, M. L. (2016). Single-sex education., Retrieved June 6, 2019, from www.oxfordbibliographies .com

Slabu, L., & Guinote A. (2010). Getting what you want: Power increases the accessibility of active goals. *Journal of Experimental Social Psychology, 46*. doi:10.1016/j.jesp.2009.10.013

Staw, B. M. (1980). The consequences of turnover. *Journal of Occupational Behavior, 1*, 53–273.

Subedi, S., Hamal, M., & Kaphle, H. P. (2013). Sexual harassment in the hospital: Are nurses safe? *International Journal of Health Sciences and Research, 3*(6), 41–47.

Talboys, S. L., Kaur, M., VanDerslice, J., Gren, L. H., Bhattacharya, H., & Alder, S. C. (2017). What is eve teasing? A mixed methods study of sexual harassment of young women in the rural Indian context. *Sage Open, 7*(1). doi:10.1177/2158244017697168

Taylor, E. A., Smith, A. B., Welch, N. M., & Harden, R. (2017). You should be flattered: Female sport management faculty experience of sexual harassment and sexism, *Women in Sport and Physical Activity Journal, 26*(1), 53–53. doi:10.1123/wspaj.2017-0158

Tecco, H., McGuinness, D., McDowell, M., Stotz, C., Tam, E., & Evans, B. (2018). Women in healthcare 2017: How does our industry stock up? *ROCKHEALTH*, https://rockhealth.com /reports/women-in-healh:Rockhealth.com

Thurston, R. (2018). Sex harassment can make victims physically sick, studies reveal. *Health Science (The Washington Post)* https://www.washingtonpost.com/national/health-science/sex -harassment-can-make-victims-physically-sick-studies-reveal/2018/02/07/1e018f3a-05f5 -11e8-b48c-b07fea957bd5_story.html?utm_term=.4913954ba479

Ton, Z., & Huckman, R. S. (2008). Managing the impact of employee turnover on performance: The role of process conformance. *Organization Science, 19*(1), L56–68.

Video Voyeurism Prevention Act. S. 1301 (108th): Video Voyeurism Prevention Act of 2004 https://www.govtrack.us/congress/bills/108/s1301/text

Wang, Q., Bowling, N. A., Tian, Q. T., Alarcom, G. M., & Kwan, H. K. (2018). Workplace harassment intensity and revenge: Mediation and moderation effects, *Journal of Business Ethics, 5*(1), 213–234. doi:110.1007/s/0551-016-3243-2

Wiktionary. Sexualism. https://en.wiktionary.org/wiki/sexualism

Witz, A. (1990). Patriarchy and professions: The gendered politics of occupational closure, *Sociology, 24*(4):675–684. doi:10.1177/0038038590024002400400

Wood, J. (2018). News: Sexual harassment and a physician's career, *Emergency Medicine News 40*, 3A–p doi:10.1097/01/EEM.0000531294.68988.66

Xin, J., Chen, S., Kwan, H. K., Chui, R. K., & Yim, F. H. (2018). Work-family spillover and crossover effects of sexual harassment: The moderating role of work-home segmentation preference. *Journal of Business Ethics, 147*(3), 619–629.

Yang, K. E., & Ham, S. H. (2017). Truancy of systemic discrimination: Anti-discrimination legislation and its effect on school attendance among immigrant children. *The Social Science Journal, 54*(2), 216–226.

Yourdictionary.com. Sexualism. https://www.yourdictionary.com/sexualism#wiktionary

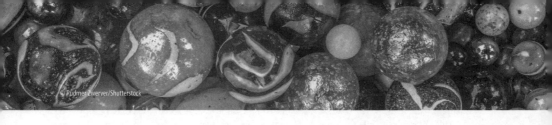

CHAPTER 4

IQism in Healthcare Workplaces and Output Maximization

"Intelligence is the ability to adapt to change."

– Stephen Hawking

LEARNING OBJECTIVES

After completing this chapter, each reader will be able to:

- Define IQism and confirm its existence in healthcare environments.
- Debate whether people of very high IQs and lower-than-average IQs are stigmatized in healthcare and other workplaces.
- Identify strategies for maximizing output for individuals in healthcare workplaces across different types of "intelligences."
- Compare and contrast strategies that all "parties" can use in order to reduce IQism as a constraint to output maximization.

▶ Introduction: Measuring Cognitive Skills

Despite the vastness of its presence, IQism continues to be unacknowledged as a phenomenon in workplaces in general. And, while **IQism** affects all human communications, some evidence exists that it may have a strong presence in healthcare workplaces. Both historically and contemporaneously, IQ has been measured by an Intelligence Quotient (IQ) test. The existence of such instrumentation is attributed to Alfred Binet and Theodore Simon who, in 1904, developed a tool for measuring cognitive skills. Introduced to the world in 1905, this test came to be known as the first "IQ test" (Minton, 1998). Over the years, this unique assessment tool has undergone many changes as a result of additional testing by other researchers. This initial IQ test has led to the development of other instrumentation to measure cognitive skills such as the Wescheler's Adult Intelligence Scale (Wescheler, 1939), the Woodcock-Johnson test (1977), and the Das–Naglieri Cognitive Assessment System (1975). Other methods of measuring cognitive capabilities have also evolved from Binet's and Simon's original intelligence scale.

Independently of the methods used to test a person's intelligence, such efforts have been controversial. Critics of the standard IQ instrumentation believe that the absence of emotional quotient (EQ) measures generates a misrepresentation of an individual's overall IQ. Moreover, researchers have discovered that a person's IQ can change (Ramsden 2011; Miller et al. 2009). Therefore, assigning an IQ number to an individual at a specific time as a measure of cognitive ability may not truly represent the person's overall intelligence. Additionally, inverse relationships occur between people with higher intelligence measurements and an inability to recall simple information. Likewise, people with lower cognitive skill measurements may simultaneously be highly evolved in selected intellectual areas. While counterintuitive, these occurrences do exist. Albert Einstein, reportedly a person with a boundary-setting IQ, allegedly would often forget information such as his phone number and/or address (Agarwal & Sen, 2014). This could be because highly intelligent people may focus on ideas and concepts rather than the domain of the mundane. Thus, the phrase "absent-minded professor" has been adopted into popular culture as evidenced by stereotypical characters in movies such as *The Nutty Professor* (1963), *Back to the Future* (1985), and the *Harry Potter* movie series (2001–2011).

But, cognitive skills are only one type of intelligence as revealed through films such as *Rain Man* (1988), *A Beautiful Mind* (2001), *Good Will Hunting* (1997), and others that illustrate this occurrence. As can be seen, the breadth and depth of the complexities associated with the concept of "high intelligence" makes it difficult to accept measured IQ as a true representation of a person's collective intelligences. However, the IQ test is still considered as the premiere testing method for human intelligence. It is highly trusted and universally used. Our society does use IQ to describe the level of a person's intelligence. This practice can, as a result, lead to IQism. The thesis in this chapter is that IQism may more often reveal itself in healthcare workplaces than in any other setting outside of educational institutions. While IQism is informally and/or formally present in all workplaces, this phenomenon may be particularly operative in healthcare workplaces.

▶ IQism in Healthcare Workplaces

In some respects, it can be argued that IQism is interwoven into virtually every area of health care. Vapiwala (2018) summarizes recent challenges in radiology because an increasing number of residents now experience difficulties in "passing" the American Board of Radiology Initial Certification. Some would argue that varied IQs determine those who pass the certification exam and those who do not.

However, the primary question raised by Vapiwala (2018) is whether the cognitive skills required to pass and succeed at the Initial Certification are directly predictive of the quality of the services that a radiologist will provide in the workplace.

Emanuel and Gudbranson (2018) also ask the implied question, "Do the medical schools that admit the highest IQ medical students produce physicians who maximally contribute to the length and quality of human lives?" Willoughby and Boutwell (2018) introduced empirical research that provides research findings regarding the role of IQ in the workplace. Their study found that the correlation coefficient between IQ and the workers' performance in the workplace is 0.65. A correlation coefficient of 0.70 and higher is considered as a strong correlation. Thus, 0.65 suggests that a relatively strong connection does exist between IQ and the maximization of workplace outcomes. Willoughby and Boutwell (2018) further argue that the necessity of advanced reasoning and problem-solving needed in medicine suggests that a high IQ is essential in this area of health care. However, they also introduce the idea that high emotional intelligence must be paired with high cognitive skills in order to achieve the maximization of outcomes in medical workplaces.

When IQ research is reviewed for people who have entered healthcare workplaces as nurses, the emphasis is not on high cognitive skills. Rather, the need for high levels of emotional intelligence is emphasized. Benson et al. (2010) measured the Emotional Intelligence of 100 nurses and confirmed that they scored within a range associated with high social intelligence. Por et al. (2011) also measured the emotional intelligence of nurses to determine the relationship between this unique workplace competency and much needed life trends such as coping and stress management. However, nurses are trained in different ways. It is not surprising that Shin et al. (2011) evaluated nurses who had an Associate of Arts degree and those with Baccalaureate degrees in nursing and identified them as possessing different cognitive skills as measured by critical thinking evaluations. This research suggests that IQism does exist in healthcare workplaces. Moreover, it operates in a way that is so subtle and so pronounced that researchers automatically assume that nurses do not have high IQs.

Moreover, when studies are conducted on IQ and healthcare administrators, a similar pattern occurs. Freshman and Rubin (2002) focus on the importance of emotional intelligence for healthcare administrators. Faguy (2012), another researcher, also completed a literature review of healthcare students and other professionals. The theme was the role of emotional intelligence. In contrast, Hauser (2002) measured IQ across a number of professions. This researcher found that physicians have IQs that exceed those of healthcare administrators. However, they found that CEOs of startups, engineers, and college professors have IQs that equal those of physicians. Accordingly, it is not surprising that IQism in healthcare workplaces delivers to physicians a level of respect and honor that may or may not support maximum workplace productivity.

IQism as a Source of Conflict in Healthcare Workplaces

Jain (2016) reports that many physicians sometimes experience negative responses from various persons in their healthcare workplaces. These adverse responses reduce workplace productivity. Unfortunately, physicians attribute the main cause of their current workplace unhappiness to healthcare administrators. Cantlupe (November 7, 2017) argues that the 3,200% increase in healthcare administrators from 1975 to 2010 versus the 150% growth in the number of physicians over the same time period has created a struggle for leadership within healthcare workplaces. Drummond (2015) describes the productivity loss that currently characterizes healthcare workplaces as a result of clashes between the physician and the administrator. One cause for such conflict is the failure of healthcare administrators to solicit, consider, and integrate physicians' views into current and proposed workplace practices. Drummond also reports on a presentation by Dr. Sachin Jain, CareMore Health System. Dr. Jain stated, "The relationship between physicians and healthcare administrators has never been more broken than it is today."

Pratt et al. (2012) also acknowledge the loss in productivity that is occurring as a result of physician/administrator conflicts. They then argue that because physicians are a large cost center in healthcare institutions, and administrators must bring down costs, physicians'/administrators' conflict is the result of a natural competition over the use of resources. Similarly, Southwick (1971), in a now-classic article, described the physicians/hospitals administrators' conflict that existed at that time as a present-day symptom of a problem that is a part of the history of the healthcare system. Baker and Baker (1999) recognized the need to reconcile ideological differences between psychiatrists and the administrators of a mental health center. These differences caused workplace dissatisfaction and high rates of turnover. Herrell (2001) described a model in which respect for family induced change. Other solutions could also be cited. However, each proposed intervention is highly dependent on the examination of the causes and magnitude of such conflict. In the next subsection, IQism is introduced as a way to not only understand physician/administrator tensions in healthcare workplaces, but also to understand tensions among other workers as well.

Understanding Workplace Interactions through the Lenses of IQism

Within the overall history of humankind, the idea of comparing human intelligence among individuals is a relatively new concept. The Binet-Simon tool (1905), the initial tool for measuring cognitive skills, was introduced as a diagnostic tool for gauging how children could be best educated (Zangwill, 1987). Since that time, IQism has developed as a set of adverse beliefs, attitudes, and behaviors towards individuals and groups based upon conclusions regarding their cognitive skills. It has extended to the assignment of labels of inferiority and/or superiority to racial/ethnic groups with people from Western and East Asia being assigned the status of being the most intelligent human subgroups on the planet (Lynn and Vanhaned, 2006).

However, IQism also operates within, as well as between, racial/ethnic groups (Chan et al., 1997). Indeed, intersectionalities occur as variabilities in IQ across male/female, racial/ethnic status, religion, geographic lines, and other factors become documented. Primary and secondary educational institutions have established special education programs that are designed for students whose measured IQs place them within the top 2.5% of the population and/or within the lower 2.5%, and/or who have other special needs that are not based on measured cognitive retention and processing skills. However, studies show that from classrooms to boardrooms and in regular workplaces, both groups often experience negative responses from those who are ± one or more standard deviations above or below the 100 points, which is the mean for most humans. A large body of research confirms this trend.

Gordon (2018) reviewed research by scholars from Purdue University who determined that approximately two-thirds of gifted students had experienced bullying by the time they reached the 8th grade. The article identified intellectual envy and fear of loss within intellectually competitive environments as some of the factors associated with these circumstances. Some of the bullying was associated with a "know-it-all" personality. Smith (2012) discovered that the reaction of more intellectually "normal" youth to their gifted counterparts was sometimes so severe that it also included cyberbullying. Pelchar and Bain (2014) confirm that the bullying of gifted and talented children does not automatically terminate at some point in the K-12 pipeline and/or by the child changing schools. Rather, it appears to be integrated into the gifted child's overall academic experience. Peterson (2006), in a study of 432 gifted students in the 8th grade, found that more than 67% had been bullied. Coleman et al. (2015) applied qualitative methodologies in order to gain entry into the lives of gifted students. They discovered that bullying was not the only adverse activity that was directed toward the gifted students. These youth were stigmatized as a consequence of their gifted talent. They were "labeled" by classmates and, in some cases, teachers and school administrators. Interestingly, they also encountered resistance to their ideas, their views, and their overall presence by other students and, in some cases, even by their teachers.

However, the experiences of special education students with intellectual and/or other disabilities also generated similar responses. Houchins et al. (2016) provide a summary of articles that confirm the bullying of special education students. These researchers also describe successful remedies for preventing and/or reducing these incivilities. Campbell (2017) found that students with autism spectrum disorder were particularly subjected to bullying in the form of physical assault, verbal abuse, and social isolation. Stated differently, IQism is directed towards persons who embody both IQ extremes. That is, assumptions of superiority and inferiority are applied to both groups of intellectually nonconforming students.

Gifted Individuals in Healthcare and Other Workplaces

While little research has been conducted, some evidence exists that IQism may follow those two groups into their respective workplaces. Nauta and Corten (2002) used case studies to show that decreased productivity due to conflicts between gifted and average-to-bright workers can occur. While Gardner and Hatch (1989) have identified **multiple intelligences** that individuals embody—bodily, verbal-linguistic, logical-mathematical, musical, naturalistic, visual-spatial, and intrapersonal, cognitively gifted individuals have an advantage in verbal-linguistic and logical-mathematical skills. Such differences suggest that gifted adults may bring traits such as those listed in **TABLE 4.1** into their workplace.

Rinn and Bishop (2015) conducted an in-depth review of the literature on gifted children who grow up and enter the workplace as gifted adults. This study revealed that not enough research has been conducted on the topic. It also

TABLE 4.1 Differential Characteristics that Gifted Adults May Bring into Healthcare and Other Workplaces

Characteristic	Potential Impact (Positive)	Potential Impact (Negative)
Greater rapidity in thinking	Earlier recognition of problems and their solutions	More thought-switching, therefore, causing others to see them as "disorganized"
Higher sensitivity that manifests itself intellectually, emotionally, imaginatively, and in other areas.	May identify areas that require strengthening by their managers that their managers have not yet observed.	Other workers may see these issues as unimportant and management may see them as "meddling."
Introversion	May exhibit higher productivity as a result of preferring to complete work rather than socialize with people.	May not participate in workplace social activities, which further separates them from the workers.
Creativity	The thought processes of the gifted and talented may be more creative and, as a result, they may craft more original approaches to the execution of assigned and unassigned work.	Colleagues may interpret these efforts as attempts to show off. Managers may be annoyed that the workers went beyond the scope of the assignment. The gifted worker may become frustrated because his or her creative vision is not "bought into" by the manager and/or colleagues.
Solutions	Because of the creativity of their thought processes, they may be more likely to quickly predict outcomes of existing work processes.	The workplace managers and employees may be unable to "buy into" the worker's creative process.
Independence	Opinions, values, and behaviors are more likely to differ from the norm of the healthcare or other workplace.	The failure to conform may be viewed as generating liabilities in the workplace rather than assets.
Overall impact	The gifted workers may feel misunderstood, overly constrained, and isolated. Thus, their potential output in the workplace may never be achieved.	Conflicts with other workers and with managers may occur and, discouraged, the workers may diminish overall workplace output.

Modified from Nauta, N. and Corten, F. (2002). Gifted adults in work, *Tijdschrift voor Bedrijfs- en Verzekeringsgeneeskunde (Journal for Occupational and Insurance Physicians)*, *10*(11), pp. 332–335.

suggests that whether gifted children grow up and maximize their output in workplaces is a function of a wide range of variables including past experience, type of occupation and/or career, and other factors. Moreover, Stambaugh and Ford (2015) imply that when giftedness in the workplace intersects with other subgroup characteristics, workplace productivity may decrease even more. Because of the perception that certain racial/ethnic or income groups fall into the lowest percentile in terms of high IQ, it is not surprising that Stambaugh and Ford discovered that gifted Americans whose origins are African and/or Latin countries, and/or Americans of any race/ethnicity whose families were low income experience additional "microaggressions." This is because the observation of "genius" in a member of a group whose genius has been previously denied generates even more animosity.

Makel et al. (2016) tracked 259 participants in Duke University's Talent Identification program from age 12 to age 40. This research confirmed that gifted children often enter the workplace as gifted workers. Approximately 37% of the group completed their doctorates and 9% were so innovative that they received patents for original products and/or processes. Similarly, a number of the youth became "…high-level leaders in major organizations." Evidence exists that conflicts occur in healthcare workplaces between individuals based on IQ and that these conflicts prevent output maximization. Rahim (2017) emphasizes the criticality of developing organizational leadership and a work style and culture that minimize workplace conflict. However, IQism as a source of conflict in healthcare and other workplaces has been largely unrecognized. A content analysis was completed by the authors of major healthcare management and human resource management textbooks. Not a single one mentioned the existence of workplace conflict based on cognitive differences in information intake, processing, and work output. Moreover, when the researchers also looked at general academic and nonacademic textbooks and general audience books on management and/ or human resources, IQism has primarily remained under-discussed. But, IQism not only involves gifted and talented individuals who have become adults, it also reduces the output of youth with cognitive disabilities who grow into adults and enter into the workplace.

Talent Management and IQism

IQism in healthcare environments operates in multiple ways. At the first level, IQism may occur because employees in health care assume that various workers have certain cognitive skills based on where they are placed in that environment. Often, it is assumed that employees who are in the C-suite (CEOs, CFOs, etc.) and physicians are the most intellectually gifted people in the workplace. Accordingly, nonphysician practitioners, nurses, social workers, and other individuals in healthcare environments are assumed to be less-gifted. Rather than assessing giftedness by years of education and position description, supervisors and managers can be trained to evaluate those reporting to them based on behaviors. Questions such as those listed in **BOX 4.1** can be asked about each worker.

Box 4.1 is designed to assist healthcare administrators and managers in identifying gifted workers across occupations in healthcare environments. However, it is also critical for healthcare administrators and managers to be introspective and

BOX 4.1 As One Doeth...Identifying Gifted Workers by Their Behavior

- Do you manage one or more workers who appear to become excited by workplace challenges?
- Do you manage workers who appear to be more productive when supervision of tasks is minimized?
- Do you have workers whose productivity is maximized when they work alone but who become embroiled in conflict and discouraged when working as a team?
- Have you observed that some workers appear to establish their own standards of work behavior for themselves and that in most of these cases, the standards exceed those of the organization?
- Do such workers routinely deliver far more than the minimum when left unsupervised?
- Do you manage workers who dislike "regular" tasks that are completed in "regular" ways but who seem happy when given the opportunity to innovatively approach work assignments?
- Do you manage workers who identify previously unobserved fragilities in their job areas?
- Do you manage workers who complete tasks more quickly and with higher quality than their peers with similar assignments?

Constructed by the authors based upon small group discussions with gifted persons.

understand whether they see gifted workers as an asset or a liability in their workplaces. **BOX 4.2** lists some questions that every healthcare administrator may wish to ask themselves.

The purpose of Box 4.2 is to encourage healthcare administrators and managers to determine their willingness to adapt to the characteristics of gifted workers. The organization, Gifted Adults Foundation (2015), provides a number of guidelines that can be adopted by current or future healthcare administrators or managers who wish to prepare themselves to more effectively maximize workplace output through the improved management of their gifted workers. **BOX 4.3** summarizes some of these recommendations.

How Gifted Workers Can Enhance Output Maximization in a Healthcare or Other Workplaces

Most outcomes reflect many interactions. Accordingly, it is easy to understand that the maximization of outcomes in the healthcare workplace may also require changes from the gifted worker. **BOX 4.4** suggests some behavioral modifications that may be necessary. While IQisms may generate an adverse response to giftedness, gifted workers are also responsible for being a co-partner. Thus, it is important that gifted workers remember their past experiences and ask, "What did I do to contribute to conflict and/or other discomfort?"

If gifted workers are true to themselves, they will see that through actions such as those listed, they do propagate actions and attitudes that reduce productivity.

BOX 4.2 Assessing My Tolerance for Managing Gifted Workers

1. I honestly have tolerance for "gifted" employees even when they are observably "different."	Strongly Agree	Somewhat Agree	Agree	Somewhat Disagree	Disagree
2. The "gifted" employees whom I encountered in the workplace were too conflictual and disagreeable for me to embrace.	Strongly Agree	Somewhat Agree	Agree	Somewhat Disagree	Disagree
3. While I have supervised individuals with extraordinary intellectual ability, their contributions to the workplace were diluted by their failure to "fit" into the overall work culture.	Strongly Agree	Somewhat Agree	Agree	Somewhat Disagree	Disagree
4. My memories of gifted people from my high school days are, on average, positive.	Strongly Agree	Somewhat Agree	Agree	Somewhat Disagree	Disagree
5. In my opinion, my managerial style allows gifted workers the freedom they need to excel.	Strongly Agree	Somewhat Agree	Agree	Somewhat Disagree	Disagree
6. While I do not micromanage, I do closely supervise my employees as part of my efforts to maintain quality control.	Strongly Agree	Somewhat Agree	Agree	Somewhat Disagree	Disagree

7. In working with gifted workers, I give them the assignment but do not try to tell them how to carry it out.	Strongly Agree	Somewhat Agree	Agree	Somewhat Disagree	Disagree
8. I ensure that my gifted workers have: 1) the freedom to introduce variety into their assignments; 2) a sufficient workload to hold their interest; and, 3) autonomy in how they complete their assignments.	Strongly Agree	Somewhat Agree	Agree	Somewhat Disagree	Disagree
9. I feel that my management style supports the creativity and innovation that gifted employees bring to the workplace.	Strongly Agree	Somewhat Agree	Agree	Somewhat Disagree	Disagree
10. Based upon my understanding of the literature on gifted workers, they absolutely love meetings because meetings provide an opportunity for planning actions in advance.	Strongly Agree	Somewhat Agree	Agree	Somewhat Disagree	Disagree
11. I ensure that I give my gifted workers as many new assignments as possible in order to prevent boredom since boredom will reduce their contributions to the workplace.	Strongly Agree	Somewhat Agree	Agree	Somewhat Disagree	Disagree

(continues)

BOX 4.2 Assessing My Tolerance for Managing Gifted Workers *(continued)*

12. Because gifted workers enjoy acquiring new knowledge, and skills, I give them assignments that other employees would consider burdensome.	Strongly Agree	Somewhat Agree	Agree	Somewhat Disagree	Disagree
13. I am sensitive to those gifted employees who prefer to produce at the same levels of other workers so that they can engage in their other creative interests.	Strongly Agree	Somewhat Agree	Agree	Somewhat Disagree	Disagree
14. I have observed that the workstyle of the gifted workers whom I have managed and/or encountered are overly perfectionistic.	Strongly Agree	Somewhat Agree	Agree	Somewhat Disagree	Disagree
15. In every environment in which I have worked as an employee or manager, gifted workers simply do not "fit in" and seeking to interface with them is a strain.	Strongly Agree	Somewhat Agree	Agree	Somewhat Disagree	Disagree
16. Most of the gifted workers whom I have encountered work better in groups when they are in a leadership role.	Strongly Agree	Somewhat Agree	Agree	Somewhat Disagree	Disagree

17. Gifted workers annoy me by asking too many questions and, in some cases, questions that are too complex to answer.	Strongly Agree	Somewhat Agree	Agree	Somewhat Disagree	Disagree
18. The gifted workers I have encountered need to learn more about the things they do in the workplace that annoy their supervisors and their colleagues.	Strongly Agree	Somewhat Agree	Agree	Somewhat Disagree	Disagree

Data from Nauta, N. and Corten, F. Gifted adults in work, *Tijdschrift voor Bedrijfs- en Verzekeringsgeneeskunde (Journal for Occupational and Insurance Physicians), 10*(11), pp. 332–335; Lubinsky, D. Benhow, C. P. and Kell, H. J. (2014). Life paths and accomplishments of mathematically precocious males and females four decades later. *Psychological Science, 25*(12), 2217–3241 and; Persson, R. S. (2009). Intellectually gifted individuals' career choices and work satisfaction: a descriptor study, *Gifted and Talented International, 24*(1), 11–24.

BOX 4.3 Managing Gifted Workers in Healthcare and Other Workplaces

- Hold candid conversations with gifted workers so that the requirements of a particular workplace can be made explicit.
- Make recommendations to your gifted workers for improving their overall "fit" within the existing and/or targeted work culture.
- Identify ways that the gifted worker may be serving as a "trigger" for workplace conflict while not asking the worker to modify essential aspects of themselves.
- To the degree possible, do not give routine, repetitive tasks to the worker independent of their position.
- Allow as much autonomy as possible within the framework of the organizational culture.
- Assign the gifted worker to a workplace that is supportive of cognitive activities.
- Do not view the gifted worker as a competitor for your authority and position as an administrator and/or manager. Gifted individuals are often internally and not externally motivated.
- Serve as a mentor to the gifted worker in making the compromises needed in order for maximum output to occur.
- Assess the individual's performance by his/her overall outcomes rather than by the processes used to achieve those outcomes.
- However, hold the gifted workers to the same deadlines and work processes as other employees

(continues)

BOX 4.3   Managing Gifted Workers in Healthcare and
Other Workplaces   *(continued)*

- When work teams are needed to complete tasks, to the degree possible, enhance outcomes by assigning gifted workers to teams with other persons with whom they appear to be compatible. And no, these individuals do not have to be equally gifted.
- If the gifted workers whom you manage are not "people persons," reduce the level of contact with the organization's patients and/or clients by using other workers as the patient/client interfaces.

Data from Nauta, N. and Corten, F. Gifted adults in work, *Tijdschrift voor Bedrijfs- en Verzekeringsgeneeskunde (Journal for Occupational and Insurance Physicians), 10*(11), pp. 332–335; Lubinsky, D. Benhow, C. P. and Kell, H. J. (2014). Life paths and accomplishments of mathematically precocious males and females four decades later. *Psychological Science 25*(2), 2217–3241 and Persson, R. S. (2009). Intellectually gifted individuals' career choices and work satisfaction: a descriptor study, *Gifted and Talented International, 24*(1), 11–24.

BOX 4.4   Guidelines for Gifted Workers in Supporting Output Maximization
in Healthcare Workplaces

- Observe your own behaviors and identify when you are behaving arrogantly and/or haughtily towards your co-workers and/or your manager.
- Take an internal inventory of feelings and beliefs and honestly determine whether your cognitive "superiority" now includes a feeling of overall superiority to the 97.5% of humanity who do not fall into your IQ range.
- Do you find yourself inwardly seething with irritation when others ask questions or make statements that you consider "dumb"?
- Do you view advanced cognitive skills as superior to the other type of "intelligences" that Gardner describes in his Theory of Multiple Intelligences?
- Do you often allow yourself to use verbal and nonverbal communications that transmits the message to others that you are a "know-it-all"?
- Are you overly critical of others without a proposed solution?
- Do you refuse to respect the authority of your manager or supervisor because you consider yourself as an "intellectual" superior?
- Do you display empathy toward your colleagues when they make errors?
- Do you prefer to do all of an assignment yourself because you mistrust the capabilities of your co-worker(s) to complete the assignment to your satisfaction?
- When you work on a team, do you share credit equally?

Compiled by the authors from discussions with healthcare managers and administrators.

Independent of the responses to the listed questions, there are some clear practices that gifted workers can follow that will allow them to engage in output maximization. **BOX 4.5** lists some of these behaviors.

There is a phrase from Luke 12:48 suggesting that for individuals to whom much has been given, much is also required (Holy Bible, n.d.). Therefore, gifted workers can also support output maximization in the workplace by delivering "much" to the success of the overall workplace. **BOX 4.6** lists some additional "responsibilities" that gifted workers may wish to consider "delivering."

BOX 4.5 Practices that Every Gifted Worker Should Demonstrate in Healthcare Workplaces

Every gifted worker should:

- Know their employer's history and all services and products.
- Correct attitudes that do not embrace a workplace commitment.
- Demonstrate strong interpersonal and communication skills including the ability to engage in active listening, to ask effective questions, and to understand management's needs.
- Use excellent verbal and nonverbal communication skills in written, face-to-face, telephonic and electronic communications while ensuring that co-workers understand the vocabulary used.
- Demonstrate emotional intelligence by "listening" to the unspoken communications of the Manager or patients.
- Remain open to criticism from the Supervisor or client/patient.
- Be willing to transmit sincerity and caring.
- Use shorter words and shorter sentences to avoid confusion.
- Deliver words with confidence but not with arrogance.
- Use concrete facts, words, and expressions rather than intellectual jargon with co-workers.
- Avoid negative words or those that may elicit strong emotional responses from co-workers or patients.
- Use words that have strength and descriptive quality, but which are, yet, sufficient.
- Tailor the words and actions to the workplace.

BOX 4.6 Additional Responsibilities of Gifted Workers

- Because gifted workers can quickly intake information, become an *Expert* regarding the services and products that your healthcare workplace offers.
- Consciously develop human relations skills and become a *Master Diplomat* in reducing tensions during encounters with angry, frustrated, and difficult coworkers.
- Use knowledge of your occupational areas to become a *Public Relations Pro* representing your healthcare area with confidence, professionalism, and critically, goodwill.
- Assist colleagues by being a *Navigator* in successfully traversing areas of difficulty that are easy for you but without making the colleague feel inadequate.
- Serve as a *Consultant* to your supervisor in identifying productivity-inhibiting practices and processing and analyzing how to best address them.
- Serve as a *Decision Maker* in making quick decisions to support output maximization.
- Finally, choose to be a *Saint* who never becomes defensive, upset, or discourteous to anyone in the workplace no matter what the provocation or situation.

IQism and "Special Education" Adults in Healthcare and Other Workplaces

While hostility and misunderstanding are sometimes aimed toward highly gifted workers, such productivity-reducing strategies are also directed toward persons who are considered below the mean in terms of cognitive skills. Beginning at the earliest point possible, it is necessary to advance enrollment, achievement, and graduation rates of special education and low-income, underrepresented students in science, technology, engineering, and mathematics (STEM), and other courses that will support their inclusion in healthcare workplaces. Since the First and Second Industrial Revolutions, it has been advancements in health sciences, engineering, chemistry, life science, geosciences, physics/astronomy, mathematics, environmental science, and, more recently, computer science and related disciplines that have catalyzed the flurry of inventive activity that has supported the nation's economic growth. Some research indicates that STEM subject matter as well as health care are easily accessible by gifted workers.

However, research on the inclusion of special education adults in healthcare workplaces is basically nonexistent in mainstream academic databases. Additionally, a look at currently funded government programs shows no initiatives that specifically target this group for inclusion in healthcare workplaces. In 2011, an estimated 13.1% of students currently enrolled in schools were special education students (Scull & Winkler, 2011). As is true for gifted and other special needs children, these students have since become adults and have entered the nation's workforce. However, even greater IQism is directed toward persons with disabilities and special needs who actually enter into healthcare and/or other workplaces. Data from the United States Department of Labor, Bureau of Labor Statistics, (Tuesday, February 26, 2019) reveal that a mere 20.6% of adults with a disability were employed as of 2018 relative to 68.6% of people without a disability. That is, people without disabilities are 233% more likely to be employed. Even when people with disabilities obtain a Bachelor's degree or higher, their labor force participation rates are only 29.8% relative to 77.1% for people with the same education who do not have a disability. Thus, a person with a Bachelors or higher college degree with no disability is 158.72% more likely to be in the workplace than their disabled counterparts. The health sector will continue to grow as the American population increases in age and as life expectancies increase. This population is an untapped and fertile future resource that can be successfully trained for employment in the healthcare industry.

Approximately 155,809,000 persons in the workforce have no disability of any type while 6,266,000 do have a disability (U.S. Dept. of Labor, Bureau of Labor Statistics, 2019). Interestingly, approximately 4.2% of people with a disability who are employed, work as healthcare practitioners and/or in healthcare technical occupations relative to 6.1% of people with no disability. Thus, people with no disabilities are 45.23% more likely to work in these areas. In contrast, as the healthcare occupations become less cognitively based, the gap in representation of people with disabilities and no disabilities varies. For example, 2.2% of people with disabilities and 2.3% of people without disabilities work in healthcare support services. In contrast, 4.4% of people with disabilities work in personal care and service occupations relative to only 3.8% of people without disabilities. Thus, people with disabilities are 15.78% more likely to work in personal care and service than people without disabilities. Approximately 5.7% of people with disabilities work in building and grounds cleaning and maintenance occupations relative to 3.7% of people with no disabilities (U.S. Dept. of Labor, Bureau of Labor Statistics, 2018). Thus, people with disabilities are 54.05% more likely to serve as cleaning and maintenance personnel in all workplaces including healthcare buildings.

Sherbin and Kennedy (December 27, 2017) discuss the status of people with disabilities and suggest that tremendous losses in workplace productivity may occur because of the number of workplaces that do not include this segment of workers. Sherbin et al. (2017), in the first known study on this subject, found that not only IQism but other types of adverse behaviors are so prevalent against children with disabilities who grow up and enter the workplace that only 3.2% of employees even self-identify to employers that they have a disability. However, approximately 30% of white collar workers have disabilities. Indeed, only 13% of this group have disabilities that can be seen, i.e., blindness, ambulatory problems, etc. Approximately, 62% of this 30% of white collar workers have intellectual disabilities, mental disabilities, illnesses, and/or other unseen conditions. The reason these conditions are not disclosed is because when known, approximately 42% of workers with disabilities discover that management and workers misjudge them and underestimate their ability to perform. The knowledge of the disability may cause management and colleagues to immediately dismiss or underestimate their current and potential contribution to the maximization of output. Approximately 31% of employees with disabilities are insulted directly by managers and colleagues. Approximately 20% report that other workers and/or their managers intentionally avoid them. Approximately 14% can feel the discomfort of others in the workplace when disabilities are known. These researchers also found that even when employees with disabilities introduce productivity-enhancing ideas into the workplace, these ideas are less well received than when they originate from employees without disabilities. The ideas from employees with disabilities are 26.31% more likely to be rejected than those from their nondisabled counterparts. Likewise, these workers are 29.54% more likely to underperform because they feel hindered by their manager and/or colleagues.

Maximizing Output by Hiring the Optimal Mix of Gardner's Intelligences

If the disability is considered intellectual or borderline intellectual, the inclusion in a healthcare workplace becomes even more unlikely. Yet, students with mild intellectual disabilities may also have a role to play in healthcare workplaces. For example, Vanderbilt University offers a Next Steps program that prepares students with intellectual disabilities for college. Think College, an organization in Boston, Massachusetts, is serving as an active agent to oversee the type of IQism that has previously kept youth with mild intellectual disabilities out of professional workplaces by keeping them out of college. George Mason University has a program called Mason Life, and UCLA also has a similar program. At some point, healthcare workplaces should decide whether such individuals fit in the American healthcare system. There is a rationale for healthcare workplaces to maximize output in healthcare environments by better managing and utilizing people with very high IQs. However, benefits may also accrue from opening the doors of healthcare workplaces to people of average or less than average IQs.

Einstein is widely credited with crafting the often-repeated quotation, "Everybody is a Genius. But, if you judge a fish by its ability to climb a tree, it will live its whole life believing that it is stupid." By contrast, Dr. Howard Gardner (1983) introduced the Theory of Multiple Intelligence and, by doing so, suggested that those who excel in logical-mathematical cognitive skills must work in conjunction with other types of "intelligences" in order to totally advance mankind. Those "other intelligences" may be physical, creative, social, emotional, and/or a range of other innate abilities that support human needs. Dr. Robert Sternberg (1985) proposed a framework that is known as **Triarchic Theory**. This theory divides human intelligence into practical skills—the strengths associated with the introduction of original approaches. Ideas and solutions is a second category. This category references the traditionally defined intelligence that characterizes those with analytic, abstract, and evaluational competencies. Perhaps it is time for healthcare institutions to collaborate with undergraduate, graduate, and professional institutions of higher education to test whether the division of labor and specialization in the field is such that there is a place for people of varied IQs.

The implication of this discussion is that human advancement has been and will continue to be slowed because human society is not and has not operated on its production possibility curve. The renowned theoretical physicist, Stephen William Hawking (2006) advanced the theory that humanity will need to populate another planet at some point to continue on a trajectory of survival. He also argued that measures are needed to prevent the growth of artificial intelligence from becoming a threat to mankind. The mathematician and self-trained biologist, Irakli Loladze (2002), based on what is now called the *Zooplankon Experiment*, argued that increased carbon dioxide in the atmosphere is increasing the production of food with less nutritional value. Arguments such as these suggest that individuals with multiple intelligences are needed in all workplaces so that the future of humankind can be saved.

▶ Summary

This chapter began by introducing the concept of IQism and documenting its operation within healthcare and other workplaces. The discussion was then expanded by identifying ways that people with extraordinary cognitive skills can be managed so that output is maximized. It is then argued that workplaces may maximize output using the optimal mix of Gardner's intelligences. Recommendations were also made regarding how healthcare workplaces can establish its optimal mix of "intelligences."

Wrap-Up

Review Questions

1. Take a minute to review your past educational and overall life experiences. Do you ever recall being annoyed by contact with other students who appear to have very high IQs? From your personal academic experiences, have you ever observed incivilities directed by others toward students who appear to have high IQs?
2. If you were a healthcare administrator or manager, what type of measures would you implement to ensure that your workplace maximizes the output of people with each of Gardener's multiple intelligences?
3. If you are assigned a group project in your graduate or undergraduate class, how could this assignment benefit from the involvement of students of multiple intelligences?

Key Terms and Concepts

IQism
Multiple Intelligences

Triarchic Theory

References

Agarwal, R. P. & Sen, S. K. (2014). Creators of mathematical and computational sciences. Springer International Publishing. doi:10.1007/978-3-319-10870-4

Baker, J. G. & Baker, D. F. (1999). Perceived ideological differences, job satisfaction and organizational commitment among psychiatrists in a community mental health center. *Community Mental Health Journal, 35*(1), 85–95.

Benson, H., Ploeg, J., & Brown, B. (2010). A cross-sectional study of emotional intelligence in baccalaureate nursing students. *Nurse Education Today, 30*(1), 49–53. doi:10.1016/j.nedt .2009.06.006

Binet, A., & Simon, T. (1905). New methods for the diagnosis of the intellectual level of subnormals. First published in *L'Année Psychologique*, 191–244.

Campbell, M., Hwang, Y-S, Whiteford, C., Dillon-Wallace, J., Ashburner, J., Saggers, B., & Carrington, S. (2017). Bullying prevalence in students with autism spectrum disorder. *Journal of Special Education, 41*(2), 101–122.

Cantlupe, J. (2017). The rise (and rise) of the healthcare administrator. Athenahealth. Expert Forum. Retrieved from https://www.athenahealth.com/knowledge-hub/practice-management/expert -forum-rise-and-rise-healthcare-administrator

Chan, D., Schmitt, N., DeShon, R. P., Clause, C. S., & Delbridge, K. (1997). Reactions to cognitive ability tests: The relationships between race, test performance, face validity perceptions, and test-taking motivation. *The Journal of Applied Psychology, 82*(2), 300–310.

Coleman, L. J., Micko, K. J., & Cross, T. L. (2015). Twenty-five years of research on the lived experience of being gifted in school: Capturing the students' voices. *Journal for the Education of the Gifted, 38*(4), 358–376. doi:10.1177/0162353215607322

Das, J. P., Kirby, J. R., & Jarman, R. F. (1975). Simultaneous and successive syntheses: An alternative model for cognitive abilities. *Psychological Bulletin, 82*, 87–103.

Drummond, D. (2015). A quality healthcare administrator? – The three commandments, https:// www.thehappymd.com/blog/a-quality-healthcare-administrator-the-three-commandments

Emanuel, E. J., & Gudbranson, B. A. (2018). Does medicine overemphasize IQ? *JAMA, 319*(7), 651–652. doi:10.1001/jama.2017.20141

Faguy, K. (2012). Emotional intelligence in health care. *Radiology Technology, 83*(3), 237–253.

Freshman, B., & Rubino, L. (2002). Emotional Intelligence: A core competency for health care administrators. *The Health Care Manager, 20*(4), 1–9.

Gardner, H., & Hatch, T. (1989). Multiple intelligences go to school: Educational implications of the theory of multiple intelligences. *Educational Researcher, 18*(8), 4–9.

Gardner, H. (1983). Frames of mind: the theory of multiple intelligences, Basic Books, ISBN 0133306143

Gifted Adults Foundation (2015). Sustainable employment of gifted workers. Insights of Positive Psychology Support Interaction with Gifted Employees at Work. Translators: Nauta, N. and van Keulen, K. https://ihbv.nl/wp-content/uploads/2014/08/IHBV-leaflet_SustainableEmployment .pdf

Gordon, S. (2018). 8 ways bullying affects gifted students. Very Well Family, https://www.very wellfamily.com.

Hauser, R. M. (2002). Meritocracy, cognitive ability and the sources of occupational success. Center for Demography and Ecology, University of Wisconsin-Madison, CDE Working Paper No. 98-07 (rev).

Hawking, S. (2006). Move to new planet, says Hawking. *BBC News.*

Herrell, J. H. (2001). The physician-administrator partnership at Mayo Clinic. *Mayo Clinic Proceedings, 76*(1), 107–109. doi:10.4065/76.1.107

Holy Bible (n.d.). Holy Bible King James Version Rembrandt Edition 1959 Library of Congress Care #59-5444. New Testament, Luke 12:48, pg. 75.

Houchins, D. E., Oakes, W. P., & Johnson, Z. G. (2016). Bullying and students with disabilities: A systematic literature review of intervention studies. *Remedial and Special Education, 37*(5), 259–273. doi:10.1177/0741932516648678

Jain, S. H. (2016). Physicians and healthcare administrators: Friends or foes? *Forbes*, https://www.forbes.com/sites/sachinjain/2016/06/29/physicians-and-health-care-administrators-friend-or-foe/#33aa44981a95

Loladze, I. (2014). Hidden shift of the ionome of plants exposed to elevated CO_2 depletes minerals at the base of human nutrition. *Ecology, Epidemiology and Global Health*, 2014; 3: e02245. Published online 2014 May 7. doi:10.7554/eLife.02245, PMCID: PMC4034684.

Lubinsky, C., Benbow, C. P., & Kell, H. J. (2014). Life paths and accomplishments of mathematically precocious males and females four decades later. *Psychological Science, 25*(12), 2217–2232. doi:10.1177/0956797614551371

Lynn, R., & Vanhanen, T. (2006). *IQ and global inequality*. Augusta, GA, Washington Summit Publishers.

Makel, M. C., Kell, H. J., Lubinski, D., Putallaz, M., & Benbow, C. P. When lightning strikes twice: Profoundly gifted, profoundly accomplished. *Psychological Science, 27*(7), 1004–1018. doi:10.1177/0956797616644735

Miller, L. J., Myers, A., Prinzi, L., & Mittenberg, W. (2009). Changes in intellectual functioning associated with normal aging. *Archives of Clinical Neuropsychology, 24*(7), 681–688. doi:10.1093/arclin/acp072

Minton, H. L. (1998). Introduction to: "The uses of intelligence tests" Lewis M. Terman (1916). In Christopher Green's Classics in the History of Pscychology. https://psychclassics.yorku.ca/Terman/intro.htm. Accessed May 20, 2019.

Nauta, N., & Corten, F. Gifted adults in work, *Tijdschrift voor Bedrijfs- en Verzekeringsgeneeskunde (Journal for Occupational and Insurance Physicians), 10*(11), pp. 332–335.

Pelchar, T. K., & Bain, S. K. (2014). Bullying and victimization among gifted children in school-level transitions. *Journal for the Education of the Gifted, 37*(4), 319–336. doi:10.1177/0162353214552566

Persson, R. S. (2009). Intellectually gifted individuals' career choices and work satisfaction: a descriptive study. *Gifted and Talented International, 24*(1), 11–24.

Peterson, J. S., & Ray, K. E. (2006). Bullying and the gifted: Victims, perpetrators, prevalence, and effects. *Gifted Child Quarterly, 50*(2), 148–168. doi:10.1177/001698620605000206

Por, J., Barriball, L., Fitzpatrick, J., & Roberts, J. (2011) Emotional intelligence: Its relationship to stress, coping, well-being and professional performance in nursing students. *Nurse Education Today, 31*(8), 855–860. doi:10/1016/j.nedt.2010.12.023

Pratt, M. G., Fiol, C. M., O'Connor, E. J., & Panico, P. (2012) Promoting positive change in physician-administrator relationships: Lessons for managing intractable identity conflicts, In Golden-Biddle & J. Dutton (Eds) Exploring Positive Social Change and Organizations. Chapter 13. Using a Positive Lens to Explore a Social Change and Organizations, Routeledge, Taylor & Francis Group, 2012.

Rahim, M. A. (2011). Managing conflict in organizations, 4th edition, New York: Routledge.

Ramsden, S., Richardson, F. M., Josse, G., Thomas, M. S. C., Ellis, C., Shakeshaft, C., … Price, C. J. (2011). Verbal and non-verbal intelligence changes in the teenage brain. *Nature, 479*, 113–116. doi:10.1038/nature10514

Rinn, A. N., & Bishop, J. (2015). Gifted adults: A systematic review and analysis of the literature. *Gifted Child Quarterly, 59*(4), 213–235. doi:10.1177/0016986215600795

Scull, J., & Winkler, A. M. (2011). Shifting trends in special education. The Thomas Fordham Institute. Pg. 1.

Sherbin, L., Kennedy, J. T., Jain-Link, P., and Ohezie, K. (2017). Disabilities and inclusion: U.S. Findings. Center for Talent Innovation: New York: NY.

Sherbin, L., & Kennedy, J. T. (2017). The Case for improving work for people with disabilities goes way beyond compliance. *Harvard Business Review*. https://hbr.org/2017/12/the-case-for-improving-work-for-people-with-disabilities-goes-way-beyond-compliance

Shin, R. K., Lee, J. H., & Kim, K. H. Critical thinking dispositions in baccalaureate nursing students. *Journal of Advanced Nursing, 2006, 56*(2), 182–189. doi:10.1111/j.1365-2648.2006.03995.x

Smith, P. K. (2012). Cyberbullying and cyber aggression. In S. R. Jimerson, A. B. Nickerson, M. J. Mayer, & M. J. Furlong (Eds.), *Handbook of school violence and school safety: International research and practice,* 93–103. New York: Routledge.

Southwick, A. F. (1971). *Physicians vs. hospitals. Hospitals, 16*;45(18), 55–9.

Stambaugh, T., & Ford, D. Y. (2015). Microaggressions, multiculturalism, and gifted individuals who are black, Hispanic, or low-income. *Journal of Counseling and Development, 93*(2), 192–201. doi:10.1002/j,1556-6676.2015. 00195.x

Sternberg, R. J. (1985) *Beyond IQ: A triarchic theory of human intelligence.* New York: Cambridge University Press.

United States Department of Labor, Bureau of Labor Statistics (February 26, 2019). Persons with a disability: Labor Force characteristics summary. *Economic News Release.* https://www.bls.gov/news.release/disabl.nr0.htm

United States Department of Labor, Bureau of Labor Statistics (February 26, 2020). Persons with a Disability: Labor Force Characteristics—2019. News Release. https://www.bls.gov/news.release/pdf/disabl.pdf

Vapiwala, N. (2018). Examining the examination: The elusive bar to determine physician competence. *Practical Radiation Oncology* (PRO) doi:10.1016/j.pro.2018.04.013

Wechsler, David. (1939). *The Measurement of Adult Intelligence.* Baltimore (MD): Williams & Witkins

Willoughby, E., & Boutwell, B. B. (2018), Importance of intelligence and emotional intelligence for physicians. *Journal of American Medical Association, 320*(2), 205. doi:10.1001/jama.2018.6278. Comment and Response in Importance of Intelligence and Emotional Intelligence for Physicians-Reply (JAMA (2018). Common on Does Medicine Overemphasize IQ?

Woodcock, R. W., & Johnson, M. B. (1977). Woodcock-Johnson psycho-educational battery. Hingham, Mass, Teaching Resources Corporation.

Zangwill, O. L. (1987). Alfred Binet, in R. Gregory, *The Oxford Companion to the Mind,* pg. 88. New York: Oxford University Press.

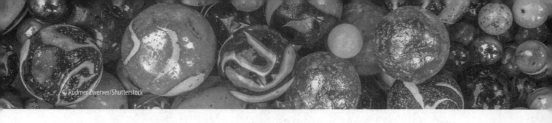

CHAPTER 5

Heterosexism in Healthcare and Other Workplaces

"The earth is the mother of all people, and all people should have equal rights upon it."

– Chief Joseph (1840–1904), the Nez Perce leader

LEARNING OBJECTIVES

After completing this chapter, each reader will be able to:

- Define heterosexism and confirm its operation in healthcare environments.
- Debate whether heterosexism operates to stigmatize some workers in healthcare and other workplaces.
- Identify strategies for addressing heterosexism so that output in healthcare and other workplaces can be maximized.

▶ Introduction: Understanding the Concept of Heterosexism

This chapter expands on previous chapters by briefly examining other subgroup-based variables that can impede workplace productivity. Evidence exists to support the idea that healthcare workplaces may not maximize output because of numerous Isms. This chapter focuses on the presence and impact of heterosexism.

A recent USA Today article (Dastagir, June 15, 2017) defined **heterosexism** as "A system of oppression that considers heterosexuality the norm and discriminates against people who display non-heterosexual behaviors and identities." Stated differently, heterosexism is the tendency for sexual behaviors based on male/female interactions to be viewed as the norm. Accordingly, lesbian, gay, bisexual, transgender, and other sexual minorities are treated in an uncivilized manner. To be clear, the labels *lesbian, gay,* and *bisexual* denote sexual preference in partners (**sexual orientation**). However, the term *transgender* describes a person who identifies with his or her non-birth gender. Conversely, the term *cisgender* describes a person who identifies with his or her birth gender. Thus, these labels describe sexual identification, not sexual orientation. However, heterosexism is associated with adverse beliefs, attitudes, and behaviors that reduce output in healthcare and other workplaces.

When the above definitions are analyzed, it becomes clear that incivilities are commonly directed against nonheterosexuals. Such collective practices are defined as heterosexism. Moreover, heterosexism is prevalent worldwide. Heterosexism exists in housing, employment, education, and other areas.

Schwegman (2018), utilizing emails designed to assess commonalities based on heterosexism, racism, classism, and nameism in 94 U.S. cities, found that heterosexism reduced overall responsiveness to same-sex couples. They also discovered that the other isms operated intersectorally with heterosexism to decrease the probability of those couples even receiving a response to their housing inquiries. Surrette (2018) completed a doctoral dissertation that analyzed the negative experiences of sexually diverse children in schools in Alberta, Canada. This researcher found that while educational policies were flexible, sexual central tendency, or heterosexism, generated adverse beliefs, attitudes, and behaviors toward gender and sexual minority students in schools. Likewise, Cech and Rothwell (2019) specifically studied the status of LGBT workers in federal agencies that are mandated to operate within the boundaries of inclusive policies. These authors found that heterosexism was prevalent to such a degree that output maximization was stifled. They also identified intersectoralities with gender, race, age, and other variables that made the impact of heterosexism more severe. This chapter focuses on heterosexism in healthcare and other workplaces.

Heterosexism in Workplaces

Increasing data reveal that workplaces globally experience reduced output based on heterosexism. This phenomenon allows the sexual preferences and the individuals' gender identifications to affect whether they will be hired. This "ism" also impacts workplace interactions and outcomes when gender minorities are hired. Ultimately, the retention, treatment, promotion, and treatment of gender minorities in the workplace is defined by heterosexism. Data from Out & Equal Workplace Advocates (2018) reveal that approximately 25% of lesbian, gay, bisexual, and transgender workers (LGBT) have experienced individual and/or organizational incivilities in American workplaces. When the gender minority is a transgender American, his or her chance of unemployment is 200% higher than the mean rate for the nation.

Other research suggest that heterosexism may be even more widespread. A 2016 survey conducted by the Center for American Progress found that over 50% of the LGBT respondents had experienced incivilities in the workplace (Singh & Durso, 2017). This same study found that some LGBT persons who were looking for a job actually changed their resumes so that there were no clues to their sexual identity because of their previous experiences with heterosexism. Independent of education level and/or years of experience, approximately 27% of transgender Americans encounter workplace conditions that prevent them from applying their knowledge and expertise toward output maximization (Out & Equal, 2018). Approximately 10% of LGBT workers resign from work because of workplace prejudice. As a result of such circumstances, as recently as 2014, approximately 25% of LGBT became poverty-stricken because of dysfunctions in the workplace. Yet, for the most part, these negative beliefs, attitudes, and behaviors have remained unaddressed.

Although legal cases on the basis of sex discrimination have been adjudicated, federal laws do not explicitly state that workplace heterosexism that results in prejudice because of personal gender choices and/or sexual orientation in general is illegal. While bills and laws have been introduced since the mid-1990s, none have passed both the House of Representatives and the Senate to become law. However, the Equal Employment Opportunity Commission does agree that discrimination based on gender choices or sexual orientation is a violation of Title VII of the Civil Rights Act of 1964. States offer even less protection (U.S. Equal Employment Opportunity Commission, 2020).

Currently, only 23 of the country's 51 states (including Washington, D.C.) have laws against the asymmetrical treatment of workers because of their gender identity or sexual orientation. Moreover, not only do a majority of the states in the United States not protect workers from the heterosexualistic treatment of gender minorities in the workplace, but 26 or 50.9% of states (including Washington, D.C.) allow workplaces to fire an employee if it is discovered that the employee is a transgender American or other sexual minority (Movement Enhancement Project, 2018). While some protection was offered to transgender individuals for a period of time, this is no longer true. Specifically, Executive Order 13672 protected transgender individuals from workplace discrimination for approximately three years before being reversed by the Department of Justice in 2017. Again, it is important to remember that "pointing fingers" and/or assigning blame regarding the "Isms" that have existed over time and space is a highly dysfunctional worldwide practice. Data from Out and Equal, reveal that 72 countries across the globe practice extreme heterosexism. That is, they maintain laws that criminalize sexualistic behaviors between individuals of the same sex. The penalties range from fines to capital punishment. However, Catalyst (June 6, 2018) reports that some improvements have been made within the United States. Approximately 91% of Fortune 500 companies do have nondiscrimination policies that are inclusive of heterosexism. Such policies support workplace output maximization.

The LGBT Population and Healthcare Workers

Brown (2017) introduces data that reveal that in addition to experiencing heterosexism in healthcare workplaces as employees, the LGBT population may be overrepresented in healthcare workplaces as consumers of healthcare services. First, the number of LGBT people in 2016 was 10.1 million individuals or 4.1% of the population based on a Gallup Poll from the Pew Research Center (June 13, 2017). This represented a 21.68% growth rate from the 8.3 million people who indicated membership in this culturally diverse group in 2012. Relative to the percentage of the overall population, the figure increased from 2.5% in 2012 to 4.1% in 2016—a 64% rate of growth. This percentage is expected to increase in the future as bias toward this group of Americans disappears. In addition, the Pew Research Center's data indicated that the greatest percentage of the LGBT population defined themselves as bisexual in 2013. In contrast, 19% self-defined as lesbians, 5% as transgender, and 36% as gay men. However, approximately 16% of the overall population were people aged 65 and older in 2018 (Census Bureau, 2019)—a group that is less likely to identify as LGBT and, as a result, may have been under-represented in surveys. However, as younger groups emerge, the number and percentage of the population who define themselves as people who are not included in the heterosexism central tendency will increase. These greater acknowledgements of personal sexual preferences may increase the presence of people who identify as LGBT in healthcare and nonhealthcare marketplaces.

The Pew Research Center's data also revealed that 4.4% of females describe themselves as LGBT relative to 3.7% of males. Thus, women are 18.92% more likely to identify themselves as a member of this gender minority. Ethnically, population growth is more prevalent among the racial/ethnic groups that have the highest proportion of LGBT people. For example, in 2010, the Asian-American population was 4.7% of the country's population and by 2016, this number had grown to 5.2% of the overall population. The June 12, 2017, report using the Pew data revealed that 4.9% of Asian Americans identify as LGBT. Latinx Americans had a population growth rate of 6.13% - from 16.3% to 17.3% during the same period. Approximately 5.4% of Latinx Americans reported that they were LGBT in the most recent Pew poll. African Americans, a group that comprised 12.6% of the population, had the third highest proportion of people who assessed their sexual preferences as being LGBT. Approximately 3.6% of White Americans who responded to the survey reported themselves as having a LGBT self-identification. Finally, approximately 5.5% of people with annual household incomes of less than $36,000, 4.0% of those with incomes from $36,000 – $89,999, and 3.7% of persons with incomes of $90,000 per year or more described themselves as part of the growing LGBT population. As these changes continue to occur, Americans who self-identify as LGBT will be increasingly represented in health care as patients and employees.

Mayer et al. (2008) assert that LGBT individuals experience a greater number of health risks than heterosexuals, the sexual majority. For example, the Centers for Disease Control and Prevention (January 25, 2017) identifies depression, tobacco, substance use, and other conditions as health risks for gay men. These researchers found that males who have sex with males are 3,900% more likely to test positive for HIV than their heterosexual counterparts. Yet, when health care is sought, factors ranging from homophobic reactions and stigma to explicit bias are often encountered in healthcare workplaces. Similarly, Huebner et al. (2015) argue that LGBT youth are at greater risk of suicide, violence, bullying, and other health risks. Hafeeze et al. (2017) had similar conclusions. As a result, this population may be over-represented among users of healthcare services.

An abundance of research reveals that high productivity does not occur when the LGBT population enters into healthcare marketplaces as consumers. Vermier et al. (2018) suggest that a disparity chain exists with multiple factors that create "... avoidance and underutilization of healthcare" (page 232). This outcome reflected the abundance of negative interactions among healthcare workers. The transgender population in this study also had greater disease and early death rates than sexual majorities. While this study was completed in Canada, it appears that healthcare workplaces globally underserve this population. Costa et al. (2016) found similar trends in healthcare workplaces in Brazil. As a result, they implemented an online intervention to reverse such conditions. In the United States, the Center for American Progress 2017 survey (Singh & Durso, 2017) also found that LGBT individuals reported having difficulty finding substitute medical care. This response reflected a reluctance to visit providers who demonstrated discrimination. Additionally, 8% of the respondents who identified as lesbian, gay, or bisexual indicated that they had experienced negative behaviors such as the outright refusal of service by a medical or healthcare provider due to the provider's heterosexual beliefs. The percentage was much higher for transgender respondents—29%. Thus, within U.S. healthcare workplaces, healthcare professionals sometimes fail to maximize output with sexual minorities. But, in a literature review, Mitchell, Lee, Green, and Skyes (2016), imply that the failure to maximize output in treating LGBT patients is not always due to implicit and/or explicit bias. Rather, they argue that the **care of these patients has not been adequately integrated into the educational programs of clinical professionals**. Healthcare professionals need clinical **training** as well as interventions to reduce the impact of adverse beliefs, attitudes, and behaviors toward this diverse population.

In a review of worldwide literature, Albuquerque et al. (2016) found that extreme explicit bias is directed toward people who do not conform to the beliefs of heterosexism by healthcare professionals. **BOX 5.1** lists a few of these findings.

While the relative experience of males and females were not compared in Box 5.1, the studies cited reveal that the services offered to lesbian women were 900% more likely to not include a pap test and 300% more likely to not include a mammogram.

A number of factors cause these circumstances in healthcare workplaces. As mentioned, one factor that reduces output maximization with LGBT patients is the fact that healthcare professionals are not given behavioral health training so that they refuse to allow their values and beliefs to be imported into the workplace.

BOX 5.1 How Workers in Healthcare Workplaces Respond to LGBT Patients

- Tremendous differences in access to health care exists between sexual majority and sexual minority populations.
- Poor provider/patient communications often characterizes the treatment of this population by workers in healthcare workplaces.
- Blatant prejudice by clinicians and other healthcare professionals exist.
- Violations of confidentiality by workers in healthcare environments occur.
- Unnecessary references to the sexual orientation of patients are made.
- Systemic, institutional, and personal discrimination in healthcare workplaces has been identified.
- Social, religious, and other environmental norms that have been imported into the healthcare workplace are applied in a judgmental manner.
- Observable feelings of repulsion when LGBT couples express their affection in healthcare workplaces have been noted.
- As a result, a greater dependence on self-medication sometimes takes place in order to avoid the stress and stigma that is encountered in healthcare workplaces.

Modified from Albuquerque, G. A., de Lima Garcia, C., da Silva Quirino, G., Alves, M. J. H., Belém, J. M., dos Santos Figueiredo, F. W., . . . de Abreu, L. C. (2016). Access to health services by lesbian, gay, bisexual, and transgender persons: systematic literature review. *BMC international Health and Human Rights, 16*(1), 2.

Albuquerque et al.'s (2016) research found that more than 50% of a group of health-care students in the United States embodied adverse responses to sexually diverse individuals based on their religious beliefs. Moreover, upto 10–12% of these future healthcare professionals literally believed that the United States should reenact laws that criminalize same-sex relationships.

Heterosexism not only operates with patients in healthcare workplaces, it also impacts prospective healthcare employees. Risdon et al. (2000) interviewed 29 gay and lesbian medical students and residents in four Canadian cities and found that the creativity and analysis that should have been directed toward workplace solutions was redirected toward coping with workplace circumstances. And, as previously discussed, neither gender minorities nor gender majorities are adequately prepared to maximize care to gender minorities upon the completion of their training. Obedin-Maliver et al. (2011) confirm that medical schools may contribute to an absence of output maximization when patients are a part of the LGBT community by not preparing medical students to treat these patients. A survey of the 133 allopathic and osteopathic medical schools that completed all aspects of the survey used by Obedin-Maliver et al. revealed that on average, only 5 hours in the entirety of the medical program addressed the needs of this subpopulation. Moreover, the median number of hours of training on LGBT treatment needs was two hours in allopathic medical schools relative to zero hours for osteopathic medical schools.

Independent of the training provided and/or the bias, LGBT individuals persevere, graduate, and enter into healthcare as workers only to continue to experience heterosexism. In a study of LGBT physicians in Croatia, Grabovac et al. (2016) found that extreme explicit bias not only existed among colleagues but also among patients. Approximately 8.8% of the 1004 participants in the survey administered by Grabovac et al. (2019) indicated that patients would refuse to be treated by a gay or bisexual physician, and 7.9% would select not to be treated by a physician who was lesbian or bisexual.

Schvey et al. (2017) found that the 1,700 family physicians in service in African military healthcare workplaces were not responsible for the care of the country's transgender active service military personnel. Approximately 94.9% of the 300 family physicians surveyed indicated that they were underprepared to provide transgender care since they had received 3 or fewer hours of training on this subject. More importantly, 52.9% of the clinicians revealed that if they had received the needed training, they would still refuse to provide the hormonal treatment that is a critical component in the transitioning process.

Heterosexism also affects males who choose to enter workplaces as nurses. Harding (2007) conducted a very interesting study. Specifically, Harding's research revealed that males who enter healthcare workplaces as nurses tend to be stereotyped as "gay." Loughrey (2008) found similar beliefs in Ireland. This research indicated that one reason for such bias is that independent of actual gender identification, nursing requires the delivery of caring services that have been historically assigned to the female gender.

Burke and White (2001) cited a 1993 survey finding on heterosexism. This research documented that lesbian physicians may have failed to maximize their output because they experienced explicit bias while receiving their medical training. While 18.5% experienced adverse beliefs, attitudes, and behaviors because of their sexual preferences while in medical school; 32.6% were targets of explicit bias in all workplaces after their completion of medical school. However, the study did reveal a downward trend in such numbers. In a more recent study, Nama et al. (2017) used a sample of 103 medical students. These researchers found that 14.6% of the sample had directly observed explicit bias against LGBT students and 31.1% has witnessed implicit bias. Approximately 48.6% of the LGBT students did not reveal their sexual orientation to other students and even fewer allowed staff physicians to know their orientation. Approximately 41.7% of the medical students were subjected to anti-LGBT comments or jokes and/or bullying by colleagues and/or other employees in the healthcare workplace.

▶ Strategies to Support Output Maximization in Healthcare and Other Workplaces Characterized by Heterosexism

Dual strategies are needed in order to maximize heterosexism-related output problems in healthcare workplaces. First, healthcare workers must be trained to address the unique needs of sexual minorities. Some progress is being made toward the inclusion of the specific needs of these subgroups via discrimination-reducing healthcare training that have been designed to address discrimination. In a Modern Healthcare article, Johnson (August 22, 2015) stated that specialized training by medical schools that focus on the needs of the LGBT community remains rare. However, the public has been more responsive. For example, the Substance Abuse and Mental Health Services Administration (SAMHSA) has training curricula that were expressly developed to support mental health and primary care personnel in the treatment of their LGBT patients. Moreover, educational institutions such as the University of California, San Francisco, and others offer guidelines and training that are designed to address the specific needs of the LGBT community.

These types of activities should improve the care that LGBT and other sexual minority patients receive. In a 2017 study, Sekoni et al. determined that improvements in the knowledge, mindsets, and behaviors of healthcare students and professionals had occurred through the use of curricula and training aimed at increasing LGBT inclusion in healthcare environments. These researchers also suggest that the continuation of the use of these or similar curricula and training will likely increase LGBT acceptance and the understanding of practices required by healthcare professionals to improve medical care provided to these subgroups. But such trainings alone are not enough to fully decrease the negative behaviors directed toward sexual minorities who are in healthcare workplaces as employees and/or as patients.

To clarify how such a conclusion is drawn, it is important to closely examine the nature and causes of this phenomenon. While a number of variations of heterosexism may be present in human society, heterosexualistic workplace incivilities can be directly explained by what we, the authors, call the *Theory of Selectivity in Adherence to Religion-Generated Ethics*. This theory argues that the following of ethical guidelines generated by religious beliefs is not absolute. Rather, the process of acceptance and dismissal is subjective and inconsistent and, as a result, persons who embody heterosexism neutralize their use of religious ethics as a basis for their beliefs. The

Theory of Selectively in Adherence to Religious-Generated Ethics can be clearly seen in the arena of sexual behavior. Newport (2017) cites data from the Gallup Poll. This data reveal that approximately 75% of U.S. residents consider themselves religious. Moreover, Saad (2017) reveals that while 75% of Americans identify as Christians, only 24% consider the Bible the "Word of God."

In American society, despite such findings, biblical passages are often quoted as the "moral" authority for heterosexism. Recent Supreme Court decisions allow differential treatment of sexual minorities based upon empirically, nonvalidated, accepted biblical statements regarding sexual behavior. Yet, interestingly, **no Supreme Court decisions have supported differential treatment of persons who violate other biblically based "standards" of sexual behavior!** To demonstrate this point, **BOX 5.2** lists biblical passages that establish "ethical" sexual behavior for those of this particular faith.

BOX 5.2 Biblically Established Standards of Sexual Behavior for the 65% of Residents of the United States who Self-Define as "Christian"

- Heterosexual sex outside of marriage appears to be biblically banned. Yet, the Theory of Selectivity in Adherence to Religion-Generated Ethics fully accepts the violation of the guidelines below for heterosexual persons:
  - 1 Corinthians 7:2
    "But because of the temptation to sexual immorality, each man should have his own wife and each woman her own husband."
  - Hebrews 13:4
    "Let marriage be held in honor among all, and let the marriage bed be undefiled, for God will judge the sexually immoral and adulterous."
  - Acts 15: 19-20
    "Therefore, my judgement is that we should not trouble those of the Gentiles who turn to God, but should write to them to abstain from the things polluted by idols, and from sexual immorality…."
  - Galatians 5:19-21
    "Now the words of the flesh are evident:
    o Sex and immorality
    o Impurity
    o Sensuality
    o Idolatry
    o Sorcery
    o Enmity
    o Strife
    o Jealousy
    o Fits of Anger
    o Rivalry
    o Dissensions
    o Envy
    o Drunkenness
    And things like these. I warn you, as I warned you before, that those who do such things will not inherit the Kingdom of God."

Pew Research Center (2019). The Holy Bible, English Standard Version Copyright © 2001 by Crossway Bibles, a division of Good News Publishers.

The inconsistent application of the guidelines effectively demonstrates that the alleged religious basis for the differential treatment of sexual minorities in and outside of the workplace clearly demonstrates that **religious guidelines are selectively applied**. Accordingly, public policies are needed that attach penalties to documented incidents of explicit bias against sexual minorities in the workplace.

However, simply creating external rules that do not allow heterosexism in the workplace is not enough. Kelly and Barker (2016) describe the six primary errors that public health professionals make in attempting to bring about change in health-related behaviors. For example, they argue that: 1) Change strategies are designed that do not reflect research findings on how behavioral change occurs; 2) It is assumed that people behave rationally; 3) The complexity of behavioral change is often oversimplified; and, 4) Other misperceptions are accepted. To address such limits, these authors suggest that behavioral change, whether directed to one's external behaviors and/or internal behaviors, has to begin with self-analysis. Thus, employees in healthcare workplaces who direct heterosexist behaviors toward those sexual minorities who are their colleagues and patients must begin by asking themselves "Why do I have these emotional responses?" If this person uses religion as the justification for such behaviors, that person must ask, "Why do I asymmetrically apply religious doctrine to "condemn" sexual minorities' behaviors while ignoring religious doctrines toward the sexual behaviors of heterosexual Americans in my workplace and beyond?"

Based on this self-analysis, individuals can then ask, "If my sexual preferences were non-heterosexual, how would I wish for my colleagues to respond in the healthcare workplaces and how would I want to be treated by the healthcare professionals whom I encounter?" Again, as with other workplace "Isms," this suggests that introspection may need to be initiated in healthcare workplaces through group therapy rather than by mere training. Such a statement does not imply that training is not a necessary and a critical tool in all workplaces. Training certainly enhances knowledge and memorization of the policies and procedures of each healthcare institution. However, training may not be the best tool to serve as a catalyst to the much-needed behavioral change process.

To support such a conclusion, some of the standard definitions of training that are found in dictionaries can be reviewed. This range of definitions of training are provided to demonstrate that the broad number of commonly accepted definitions explicitly reveals that **training is not and was never meant to serve as a tool of behavioral change**. Yet, training appears to be the primary tool used by administrators and managers in healthcare and nonhealthcare workplaces to address the various "isms" that may be operative. Part of the reason therapeutic interventions have not yet been standardized to reduce the adverse impact of Isms in the workplace is because the American Psychological Association does not recognize hate crimes as an active explicit bias, nor other such behaviors as "behavioral health problems." Yet, while current definitions of behavioral health do not include the impact of negative beliefs, attitudes, and behaviors directed toward others as a behavioral health "problem" at this point, ample research confirm that those factors do adversely impact health.

Barsade (2002) specifically tested how negative emotions (independently of the source) affect the individual and groups in workplaces by using an experiential design. Specifically, individuals were trained to bring unpleasant moods, adverse attitudes, and other socially unacceptable responses to the workplace as part of an experiment. These responses resulted in a ripple effect that was equivalent to the introduction of a virus into a group of individuals within a closed workplace. Put another way, a process of what the author called "emotional contagion" occurred that negatively affected the functioning of the workplace. Importantly, the experiment had the same impact when the emotions introduced were positive. Both individual and group processes were elevated in these workplaces when positive emotions were introduced. But, as the list of training definitions provided in **BOX 5.3** reveal, **training cannot deliver outcomes that alter emotional contingencies**. Only behavioral change interventions can effectively change negative behaviors in the workplace that are associated with heterosexism. Only then can high productivity be achieved. A number of studies support such a conclusion.

For example, Bolte et al. (2003) examined the relationship of positive and/or negative emotions on cognitive activity. These researchers demonstrated the impact of positive and negative emotional states on reasoning by conducting an experiment involving the ability to reason using various work patterns. Substantial differences in outcomes occurred between the participants' ability to discern these work patterns based on mood. People who were in a positive mood performed at an even higher level than people in a neutral mood. Those in a bad mood performed at a lower level. Again, this study suggests that heterosexism in a workplace is a behavioral condition that, because of its impact on mood, can negatively impact the work output.

Research helps to form a hypothesis regarding the role of **serotonin**. Carver et al. (2009) suggest that employees' behavior in workplaces and/or in other life settings may be responsive to serotonergic functioning. Eating nuts, red meat, selected types of poultry, and cheese provide our bodies with tryptophan. Serotonin is known as a "feel good" chemical that the body produces. Low levels of serotonin have been linked to anxiety, fatigue, Seasonal Affective Disorder (SAD), and other mood-related conditions (Gupta et al. 2013; Meeusen et al. 2006; Gibson, 2008, Mirza, 2015). SAD can be caused by a lack of sunlight, which can result in reduced levels of serotonin (Nørgaard et al. (2017). People take serotonin supplements to lift their moods. Serotonin also induces sleep (McGinty, 2009).

Carver et al. (2009) suggest that people with low serotonin levels may be more reactive and impulsive while people with higher levels of serotonin may be more reflective. We use this finding to conclude that greater reflectivity may be associated

---

BOX 5.3   Commonly Used Definitions of the Word "Training"

- *Definition of 'Training' from Cambridge Dictionary*, www.dictionary.cambridge.org, © Cambridge University Press. Used with permission.
  "The process of learning the skills you need to do a particular job or activity" | "When you are in training for a competition, you exercise in a way that prepares you for it."
- *YourDictionary.com* (https://www.yourdictionary.com/training):
  "…the process of being conditioned or taught to do something, or the process of learning and being conditioned."
- *Longman Dictionary of Contemporary English* (https://www.ldoceonline.com/dictionary/training):
  "The process of teaching or being taught the skills for a particular job or activity."
- *Princeton's WordNet* (http://wordnetweb.princeton.edu):
  "preparation, grooming, (activity leading to skilled behavior)."

Constructed by the Authors from the sources listed.

with a reduced probability of adopting heterosexism (and/or other isms). Stated differently, there is a possibility that eating certain foods that are rich in tryptophan may increase individuals' inclination to think and reason regarding the cause and effect of their own negative behaviors.

Research on human behavior also suggests that people who have been affected by heterosexism may need behavioral counseling as part of "healing" from the trauma of their adverse experiences. Researchers such as Szymanski (2011) and Goodwin (2014), for example, describe the impact of these experiences on a person's life. However, other research also lead to the conclusion that an effort must be made to "forgive" past negative experiences. We draw this conclusion from research by Kensinger (2009), who, in a study of the relationship between emotion and memory, found that a very interesting trend exists. Specifically, memory has the power to enlarge experiences. However, this "enhancement" effect is greater with negative past experiences than with positive ones. This suggests that behavioral interventions are needed that can help sexual minorities avoid bringing the "emotional weight" of past experiences into new healthcare and/or other workplaces. Again, such a concern cannot be addressed by training alone. Rather, behavioral interventions are also needed by those who have experienced heterosexism.

Of equal interest, current and past research indicate that behavioral change is easier than is often believed. Wilson and Gilbert (2005) argue that human behavior is subject to a set of responses that they call, *impact bias*. Impact bias references individual responses to events that occur within a person's present and future lives. These authors argue that homosapiens often engage in "...*over-estimating the intensity and duration of their emotional reactions to such events*" (page 131). However, these researchers also argue that **individuals underestimate their own ability to cope with and "heal" from past events**. Again, behavioral interventions can be useful in helping people to call upon their own strength. These theories support that training alone is not enough to address heterosexism and other Isms in healthcare and other workplaces. Rather, active and prolonged **interventions** are needed.

Interventions are needed to help employees understand that behavioral change is necessary and to assist in catalyzing each individual to: 1) Confront the possibility that there may be a need to change; and 2) To assist the individual in taking the first steps that will allow needed internal change processes to become activated. For example, Kok, Peters, and Ruiter (2017) describe how *Intervention Mapping* can be used outside of its original field, promotion. Using a social ecological framework that goes beyond the individual to embrace all external and internal behavioral influences, the Intervention Mapping Approach involves several steps. First, an assessment of need must be conducted in the targeted healthcare workplace. Using quantitative and qualitative methodologies, the healthcare administrator or manager would need data that can answer the questions: "Does heterosexism operate in our healthcare environment among employees and/or between employees and patients who are sexual minorities?" Based upon the findings, the assessment process would also seek to ascertain the magnitude of heterosexism. Second, the healthcare workplace would, as part of the assessment, analyze the findings to identify the specific segments of the workforce that embody heterosexism and the nature of the causative factors and implicit and explicit premises that support heterosexist behavior. Third, based on the findings from the descriptive and causative data collection and analysis process, the Intervention Team would complete research on behavioral change interventions that can be instituted in the workplace. While evaluating interventions, the Intervention Team would consider the culture of their healthcare organization, how heterosexism operates within specific units and divisions, and other factors specific to a particular healthcare work environment.

A range of interventions are available to healthcare managers and human resources managers for use in ameliorating such Isms. Cramwinckel, Scheepers, and van der Toorn (2018) cite some of the interventions that may prepare people in healthcare and other workplaces for the introspection needed to affect behavioral change. Specifically, these authors cite research that shows the value of *edutainment* as an effective strategy for generating the introspection that is a necessary prerequisite to behavioral change. **BOX 5.4** cites some of the research findings on edutainment interventions that have initiated some change regarding heterosexism.

Other supports may also be necessary. Meis and Kashima (2017) conducted research that reveals that well-designed signage can bring about behavioral change. For example, signage that states, "When I look at you… I…see… me!!!" can be used. The constant exposure to visual images addressing key "Isms" in the workplace can, over time, support internal change.

One underused strategy by public health professionals and healthcare administrators in seeking to generate behavioral change and not merely knowledge change is *edutainment*. The current paradigm in health communication is using media to deliver health messages via public service announcements (PSA) and/or other direct communications. However, the impact of this approach is limited.

Esmaeilpour et al. (2018) have developed the idea that healthcare messages can be integrated into children's entertainment that will support behavioral changes in

---

BOX 5.4 Heterosexism Interventions That Can Be Adopted for Use in Healthcare and Other Workplaces

- The viewing of films that are inclusive of storylines regarding sexual minorities can serve as triggers for the process of behavioral change (Case & Stewart 2010).
- Moreover, it appears that individuals may be more responsive to indirect interventions than to a direct intervention considering that the research demonstrated the greater effectiveness of fiction-based rather than nonfiction interventions (Fong et al. 2015).
- Encouraging subject-related fiction reading in general appears to be an intervention that reduces adopting ideologies of superiority and inferiority (Fong et al. 2015).
- Participation in video games in which the "groups" help to cause greater acceptance of diverse subgroups in general can generate behavioral change (Adachi et al. 2015).
- Games, rather than training or "lecturing," are more effective in triggering behavioral change.
- Attempting to reduce heterosexism by discussing biological factors does not trigger a process of behavioral change (Hegarty 2010).
- Whether the focus is heterosexism or some other type of cultural diversity issue in the workplace, the provision of training that simply generates a better understanding of the specific ism has little chance of serving as a trigger for behavioral change (Bezrukova et al. 2016).

Modified from Cramwinckel, F. M., Scheepers, D. T., van der Toorn, J. (2018). Interventions to reduce blatant and subtle sexual orientation and gender identity prejudice (SOGIP): Current knowledge and future directions. *Social Issues and Policy Review*, 12(1), 183–217.

terms of the food choices that are selected by children. Wolfensberger et al. (2019) used a randomized control experiment to compare the impact of a traditional Standard Precaution Manual and an edutainment video on the same topic. These researchers discovered that the video yielded higher knowledge scores and greater satisfaction. Oduarn and Nelson (2019) carefully recorded the effectiveness of a television series as an HIV/AIDS intervention in South Africa. Kurtovich et al. (2010) assessed the impact of a PSA campaign to increase knowledge of Medicaid Managed Care in Maryland. Awareness remained low. Beaudoin (2009) assessed the outcomes of a PSA campaign to reduce post-traumatic stress disorder (PTSD) after Hurricane Katrina. Although some positive outcomes occurred, PTSD levels were unaffected. Other studies can also be cited that demonstrate that media is not being maximized as a means of health promotion that can definitively change behavior.

Yet, the power of media and entertainment as tools that can affect behavior is continually "proven" through studies on the *negative* impact of media. Harrison and Cantor (1997), in a study of 4,222 college students, argued that media use by women is associated with "disordered-eating" symptoms. Slater and Hayes (2010) found that strong evidence existed regarding the relationship between teenage smoking and certain types of media exposure. Such studies reveal that if media and entertainment can be used negatively and for behavior formation, it can also be used more positively if public health professionals shift from the PSA paradigm that is currently used and begin to explore the health communication opportunities that are natural to media and entertainment. For example, Dutta-Bergman (2006) suggests that unlike other countries, soap operas are underutilized in the United States for health communications that promote behavior change. Thus, for almost two decades, edutainment has been used to impart health communications to TV viewing audiences in some countries.

Freimuth and Quinn (2004) report that this form of health communication has been successful especially among minority viewers. Moreover, in the CDC's analysis of the 2000 *Porter Novelli Healthstyles Survey*, it was revealed that over 50% of TV viewers interviewed for the study indicated that they had gained knowledge regarding prevention information, or other characteristics of a specific disease (CDC, 2001) via television. Moreover, more than 50% of the Latinx women, African American women, and African American men who tuned in to the TV show regularly reported increased knowledge regarding a specific health issue or disease that was featured on the show. Many of the viewers also shared health information with family and friends (CDC 2001). However, as is known, the number of soap operas and non-reality TV shows aired in the United States has declined considerably over the past decade.

Read and Shortell (2011) suggest that health communication messages delivered through interactive games are a form of media that is rarely used. However, the area of edutainment has been gathering momentum as evidenced by the *12th International Conference on E-learning and Games*, which was held in Xian, China, in June, 2018. Thus, healthcare workplaces can contribute to a paradigm shift in heterosexism by demonstrating the efficacy of an alternative use of media to support both knowledge and behavioral change that can enhance productivity.

To do so, a continuum of health communications that ranges from education to edutainment is needed. As part of the effort to reduce heterosexism in healthcare workplaces, public health researchers and practitioners do agree that the health communication products and dissemination strategies must reflect the culture, values, and language of the targeted audiences (Horodynski, 2011). The health communications that are directed toward healthcare workers must be written using the unique language subtleties and subcultural tastes and preferences of the target audiences without perpetuating stereotypes. Gollust, Lantz, and Ubel (2010) discuss some complications associated with audience-specific images and behaviors. Nevertheless, the efficacy of edutainment materials must contain the language, style, cultural values, folkways, and mores of the target audience. Accordingly, revised methods must be used that bypass the current reliance on training alone.

It is commonly understood that health communications in the form of health education have the power to change health knowledge. For example, Rocha-Goldberg et al. (2010) tested a group education intervention to increase knowledge and use of the evidence-based Dietary Approaches to Stop Hypertension (DASH) diet and to increase physical activity. While progress was made, the changes were not statistically significant. However, far less research has been conducted on the efficacy use of entertainment as a tool to deliver accurate and effective information that can lead to behavioral change. Yet, enough evidence exists to support the possibility that behavioral change can occur. Lee et al. (2011), for example, developed an animated series for web dissemination regarding health disease risks. The study found that using images in addition to text had a positive effect on changes in dietary behavior within 2 weeks after viewing.

In contrast, Jackson et al. (2011), using "a randomized clinical trial research approach," hired a trained actor to deliver health communications through a DVD effort called, "Video Doctor" and obtained excellent results. Researcher Carol Cox (2008) used media for positive health purposes through "Good for You TV." However, edutainment as a health promotion strategy extends beyond television to include any form of entertainment or partial entertainment for the purpose of communicating healthcare messages. Clifford et al. (2009) tested such an approach by assessing the impact of a cooking show as a tool for increasing health knowledge and improving dietary behavior. While health knowledge relative to diet increased, dietary behavioral change did not occur ($p < 0.04$). However, Parry (2011) reported quite different outcomes. Using an historical approach, the author argued that the entire health communication campaign regarding birth control occurred through an education entertainment approach. Additionally, Jana et al. (2015) describe a successful multimedia HIV/AIDS edutainment campaign entitled OneLove that ran in Africa. It disseminated information through branded written materials that featured a slogan and logo, radio spots, and a television film series. However, an assessment that involved the *OneLove campaign* conducted by Hutchinson et al. (2012) revealed significant negative results in certain areas even though the campaign as a whole had a positive effect on the behaviors of its audience. These findings indicated that both the type of intervention as well as the dosage both affect the future behavior choices of the audience members.

Buckner-Brown and Agho (2005) analyzed HIV/AIDS PSAs that were produced and aired by the Centers for Disease Control and Prevention and the National Institute on Drug Abuse. These PSAs targeted high-risk sexual behaviors. Their use successfully altered health knowledge but did not cause behavioral change. However, emerging research now reveals that entertainment is a communication strategy that can create behavioral change. Orozco-Olvera et al. (2019) document the effectiveness of edutainment in motivating youth to embrace safer sexual practices. However, while costs and other barriers exist to using television or film as vehicles to deliver entertainment-based healthcare messages, digital technology has reduced production costs significantly and online broadcast opportunities now allow access to any target audience. Thus, telehealth products that represent nontraditional health education, edutainment, or traditional entertainment options with health messages can be disseminated to select audiences without the traditional "green-lighting" process that limited audience access in the past (Shuldman, 2010).

Walsh (2005) used the term "edutainment" because many computer games that children play deliver more than entertainment. They are a way to enhancing factual knowledge as the game is being played. Dway et al. (2015) report positive results for the delivery of health education regarding the importance of early childhood immunizations to mothers in villages via entertainment messages that were loaded onto their electronic tablets. However, Zeedyk et al. (2003) presented a detailed discussion of the results of an intervention with a comparison group that revealed the possible limitations of edutainment. Using 60 families assigned to the experimental groups and 60 families who were participants in the control group, the test of the edutainment concept revealed that although parents in the intervention reported positive outcomes, no significant ($p < 0.05$) behavioral outcomes occurred. Thus, workplaces that seek to address heterosexism in the marketplace need to carefully measure outcomes. The subsection that follows describes how edutainment-based, heterosexism interventions can be measured.

The following section, although quite technical, is included so that a healthcare administrator or human resources manager will be familiar with at least one appropriate statistical methodology before working with a statistician to perform an analysis of the success of the heterosexism edutainment intervention.

Measuring the Impact of a Workplace Edutainment Heterosexism Behavioral Change Intervention: One Recommended Approach

Data collection is the first step in an intervention of this type. Peterson et al. (2017) identified a number of tools that can be used to measure heterosexism in a healthcare and/or other workplace. Additionally, workplaces with effective grievance processes can supplement such measurements with historic data. This preliminary data can then be used to track behavior and attitude changes throughout the edutainment intervention. The baseline data collected should be expanded to include demographic, psychographic, and life experience research on each participant. Data should be collected on a monthly basis over the course of the education intervention.

Healthcare workers who engage in a heterosexism workplace intervention must choose to voluntarily participate or be recruited through outreach. A Table of Random Numbers can be used to assign participants to intervention and comparison groups. These groups would consist of at least 20+ persons each (or a higher to allow for attrition). Although the healthcare workplace intervention will take place over 6 weeks, participants should be tracked for 18 months.

Both intervention and comparison groups will require traditional, educational training using a heterosexism training modular course. The percent or proportion of participants whose heterosexism, when analyzed at the end of the intervention, reveal a downward trend would be bounded to intervals between 0 and 1. The proportion can be transformed into a logic function or log odds transformation. This transformation can then be used as the response variable in the analysis. Thus, model parameters can be exponentiated and interpreted on the effect of the odds of a decreased mean for adverse responses.

While such an approach is highly statistical, all healthcare administrators and public health and clinical students are required to take statistics. As a manager in a healthcare workplace, a statistician can be contracted. Nevertheless, the interprofessional background of a healthcare manager needs to have a working knowledge of statistics to be able to communicate with the statistician. Thus, this section is critical because it provides a robust data analysis strategy that can be used to evaluate the outcome of an intervention to reduce heterosexism in healthcare workplaces.

Specifically, the healthcare administrator will need to establish whether the edutainment intervention resulted in a decrease in the mean rate of negative responses during the study period. To assess this, two interrupted time series regression analyses using maximum likelihood estimation can be completed for each outcome using the time series data on knowledge change, willingness to change, and other measures for the comparison group and for the intervention group. The study would theorize that the variables will remain constant or slightly increase for the comparison group. In contrast, the time series data for the intervention group would remain flat at preintervention but would increase more than that of the comparison group over the intervention period.

Based on the study's exact hypothesis, an interrupted time series model with a ramp variable equaling zero during the preintervention period and equal to 0 to 17 for each of the 17 consecutive months of the intervention period would have the best fit for the intervention group. This model would have positive change but a nonsignificant coefficient on the ramp variable for the comparison group. This step in the time series analysis would involve first testing whether it remains constant or trends and seasonality using the Dickey-Fuller tests for trend and seasonality and then examining the graphs of the time series data. Since some trending is expected for both the comparison group and the intervention group, testing for trending should be conducted for both groups.

Subsequently, the data can be tested for autoregressive and moving average (ARMA) processes using the auto-correlation function (ACF), the inverse and partial auto-correlation functions (IACF and PACF), and the Ljung-Box test for white noise. The order of the ARMA term can be identified using the Extended Sample Auto-correlation Function (ESACF), the Minimum Information Criteria (AIC), and the Schartz Bayesian Criteria (SBC). Other forms of the interrupted or intervention models can be compared with the ramp model to determine the best fitting model. These options would include models that reflect a gradual, but permanent, change in heterosexism levels, an abrupt but permanent change in the key measurement variables, or models with changes in the level and slope of the change and change functions. The models for the intervention groups with significant parameter estimates would be chosen as the final models. These models would then be applied to data from the comparison group so that the impact of the edutainment intervention upon parameter estimates can be determined.

This evaluation of the outcomes of the intervention would have several limitations. First, for smaller healthcare workplaces, the sample sizes would be small.

However, the repeated measures design would offset this problem. However, measures would be necessary to prevent drop-out rates greater than 20% and to ensure that the sample sizes never fall below 10. The second challenge of the study would ensure that the allocation method is not biased. Using a random number table would reduce this risk. Through such analytical processes, any healthcare environment would be able to test whether the selected edutainment intervention was "successful." (The described methodology can be made more intelligible to a current or future healthcare manager and/or administrator via resources throughout the web to support understanding the proposed methodology.) The proposed edutainment intervention will rigorously assess any intervention other than a one-time didactic training. As long as data are collected over time using the selected instrument, this approach could be applied.

The healthcare administrator or manager could not complete this assessment directly. He or she would contract with a statistician to apply this and/or other robust statistical methodologies. Again, the description of the described approach was included to ensure that the healthcare administrator or manager who authorized the analysis has familiarity with at least one appropriately designed statistical method.

▶ Summary

This chapter provides an overview of heterosexism, another "Ism" that can impede output maximization in a healthcare or other workplace. It also provides detailed recommendations for reshaping the operation of this well-documented phenomenon.

Wrap-Up

Review Questions

1. Based on your review of heterosexism, why does it warrant a separate chapter from sexualism?
2. Conduct research that helps you assess whether output maximization in healthcare workplaces would be more diminished by negative behavior based on heterosexism that are directed toward patients and/or heterosexism-based incivilities that are directed toward healthcare employees.
3. Even if you have never had a statistics course, conduct a literature review on empirical articles on heterosexism in healthcare workplaces. Use Google to help you compare and contrast the methods used to conduct the analysis.

Key Terms and Concepts

Edutainment
Heterosexism
Intervention

Sexual Orientation
Training

References

Adachi, P. J. C., Hodson, G., Zanelle, S., & Willoughby, T. (2015). Brothers and sisters in arms: Intergroup 69 Cooperation in a violent shooter game can reduce intergroup bias. *Psychology of Violence, 5*, 455–462.

Albuquerque, G. A., Garcia, C. L., Quirino, G. S., Alves, M. J. H., Belém, J. M., Figueiredo, F. W. S., ... Adami, F. (2016). Access to health services by lesbian, gay, bisexual, and transgender persons: Systematic literature review. *BMC International Health and Human Rights, 16*(2), doi:10.1186/312914-015-0072-9

APT Academic Solutions. http://www.aptacads.com/training.htm. Accessed June, 2019.

Barsade, S. G. (2002). The ripple effect: Emotional contagion and its influence upon group behavior. *Administrative Science Quarterly, 47*(4), 644–675, doi:10.2307/3094912

Beaudoin, C. E. (2009). Evaluating a media campaign that targeted PTSD after hurricane Katrina. *Health Communication, 24*(6), 515–523. doi:10.1080/10410230903104905

Bezrukova, K., Spell, C. S., Perry, J. L., & Jehn, K. A. (2016). A meta-analytical integration of 40 years of research on diversity training. *Psychological Bulletin, 142*(11), 1227–1274.

Bolte, A., Goschke, T., & Kuhl, J. (2003). Emotion and initiation: Effects of positive and negative mood on implicit judgements of semantic coherence, *Psychological Science, 14*(5), 416–421. doi:10.1111/1467-9280.01456

Brown, A. (June 13, 2017). 5 Key findings about LGBT Americans, *FACTTANK: News in the Numbers*, Pew Research Center, http://www.pewresearch.org/fact-tank/2017/06/13/5-key-findings-about-lgbt-americans/

Buckner-Brown, J., & Agho, A. O. (2005), An examination of U.S. federally funded television public service announcements (PSAs) in changing aids risk behaviors in African American populations. *Race, Gender, and Class, 12*(3/4), 120–138.

Burke, B. P., & White, J. C. (2001). The well-being of gay, lesbian, and bisexual physicians. *Western Journal of Medicine, 174*(1), 59–62.

Cambridge Dictionary Training. https://dictionary.cambridge.org/us/dictionary/english/training

Carver, C. S., Johnson, S. L., & Joormann, J. (2009). Two-mode models of self-regulation as a tool for conceptualizing effects of the serotonin system in normal behavior and diverse disorders. *Current Directions in Psychological Science, 18*(4), 195–199. doi:10.1111/j.1467-8721.2009.1635.x

Case, K. A., & Stewart, B. (2010). Changes from diversity courses student prejudices and attitudes toward heterosexual privilege and any marriage. *Teaching of Psychology, 37*, 172–177.

Catalyst (June 17, 2019). Lesbian, gay, bisexual, and transgender workplace issues. Knowledge Center. https://www.catalyst.org/knowledge/lesbian-gay-bisexual-transgender-workplace-issues

Cech, E. A., & Rothwell, W. R. (2019). LGBT Workplace inequality in the federal workforce: intersectional processes, organizational contexts, and turnover considerations. *Industrial and Labor Relations Review*, doi:10.1177/0019793919843508

Centers for Disease Control and Prevention (2001). Gateway to Health Communication & Social Marketing Practice. 2000 Porter Novelli Healthstyles Survey. Primetime Viewers and Health Information. http://medbox.iiab.me/modules/en-cdc/www.cdc.gov/healthcommunication/toolstemplates/entertainmented/2000Survey.html

Centers for Disease Control and Prevention. Gay and Bisexual Men's Health, (January 25, 2017). For your health recommendations for a healthy you. https://www.cdc.gov/msmhealth/for-your-health.htm

Clifford, D., Anderson, J., Auld, G., & Champ, J. (2009). Good grubbin': Impact of a TV cooking show for college students living off campus. *Journal of Nutrition Education and Behavior, 41*(3), 194–200. doi:10.1016/j.jneb.2008.01.006

Collins English Dictionary. Sexual Identity. https://www.collinsdictionary.com/us/dictionary/english/gender-identity

Collins English Dictionary. Training. https://www.collinsdictionary.com/us/dictionary/english/training

Costa, A. B., Pase, P. F., de Camargo, E. S., Guaranha, C., Caetano, A. H., Kveller, D., ... Narki, H. C. (2016). Effectiveness of a multidimensional web-based intervention program to change Brazilian health practitioners' attitudes toward the lesbian, gay, bisexual and transgender population. *Journal of Health Psychology, 21*(3), 356–368.

Cox, C. (2008). "Good for You TV": Using storyboarding for health-related television public service announcements to analyze messages and influence positive health choices. *Journal of School Health, 78*(3), 179–183. doi:10.1111/j.1746-1561.2007.00282.x

Cramwinckel, F. M., Scheepers, D. T., & van der Toorn, J. (2018). Interventions to reduce blatant and subtle sexual orientation- and gender identity prejudice (SOGIP): Current knowledge and future directions. *Social Issues and Policy Review, 12*(1), 183–217.

Dastagir, A. E. (June 15, 2017) LGBTQ definitions every good ally should know. *USA Today.* https://www.usatoday.com/story/news/2017/06/15/lgbtq-glossary-slang-ally-learn-language/101200092/

Dictionary.com. Training. https://www.dictionary.com/browse/training

Dictionary Google, Training. https://www.google.com/search?ei=ZLheXdP6Eobc-gS0qaKYBw&q=google+dictionary&oq=google+dictionary&gs_l=psy-ab.3..0i131i67j0l9.3655.7673..7935...1.2..0.85.1226.17......0....1..gws-wiz.....10..0i71j35i39j0i131j0i67j0i10.-jgJs1FHlyQ&ved=0ahUKEwjTvOKI6ZbkAhUGrp4KHbSUCHMQ4dUDCAo&uact=5#dobs=training

Dutta-Bergman, M. J. (2011). A formative approach to strategic message targeting through soap operas: Using selective processing theories. *Health Communication, 19*(1), 11–18.

Dway, N. S., Soonthornworasori, N., Jandee, K., & Kaewkungwal, J. (2016). Effects of edutainment on knowledge and perceptions of Lisu mothers about the immunisation of their children. *Health Education Journal, 75*(2), 131–143. doi:10.1177/0017896915569086

Esmaeilpour, F., Hanzaee, K. H., Mansourian, Y., & Khounsiavash, M. Children's food choice: advertised food type, health knowledge and entertainment. *Journal of Food Products Marketing, 24*(4), 476–494. doi:10.1080/10454446.2017.1315843

Fong, K., Mullin, J. B., & Mar, R. A. (2015). How exposure to literary genres relates to attitudes toward gender roles and sexual behavior. *Psychology of Aesthetics, Creativity, and the Arts, 9,* 274–285. http://psycnet.apa.org/record/2015-17772-001 doi:10.1037/a0038864

Free Dictionary. Training. https://www.thefreedictionary.com/training

Freimuth, V. S., & Quinn, S. C. (2004). The Contributions of Health Communication to Eliminating Health Disparities. *American Journal of Public Health, 94*(12), 2053–2055.

Gibson, E. L. (2018). Tryptophan supplementation and serotonin function: Genetic variations in behavioural effects. *The Proceedings of the Nutrition Society, 77*(2), 174–188. doi:10.1017/S0029665117004451

Gollust, S. E., Lantz, P. M., & Ubel, P. A. (2010). Images of illness: How causal claims and racial associations influence public preferences toward diabetes research spending. *Journal of Health Politics Policy and Law, 35*(6), 921–959. doi:10.1215/03616878-2010-034

Goodwin, E. L. The long-term effects of homophobia-related trauma for LGB men and women. (2014). *Counselor Education Master's Theses,* 160. http://digitalcommons.brockport.edu/edc_theses/160

Grabovac, I., Mustajbegović, J., & Milošević, M. (2016). Are patients ready for lesbian, gay and bisexual family physicians – A Croation study: Igor Grabovac. *European Journal of Public Health, 26*(1). doi:10.1093/eurpub/ckw173.006

Gupta, A., Sharma, P. K., Garg, V. K., Singh, A. K., & Mondal, S. C. (2013). Role of serotonin in seasonal affective disorder. *European Review for Medical and Pharmacological Sciences, 17*(1), 49–55.

Hafeez, H., Zeshan, M., Tahir, M. A., & Jahan, N. (2017). Health care disparities among lesbian, gay, bisexual, and transgender youth: A literature review. *Cureus, 9*(4), e1184. doi:10.7759/cureus.1184

Harding, T. (2007). The construction of mean who are nurses as gay. *Journal of Advanced Nursing, 60*(6), 636–644. doi:10.1111/j.1365-2648.2007.04447.x

Harrison, K., & Cantor, J. (1997). The relationship between media consumption and eating disorders. *Journal of Communication, 47*(1), 40–67.

Hegarty, P. (2010). A stone in the soup? Changes in sexual prejudices and essentialist beliefs among British students in a class on LGBT psychology. *Psychology and Sexuality, 1*(1), 3–20.

Horodynski, M. A., Baker, S., Coleman, G., Auld, G., & Lindau, J. (2011). The Healthy Toddlers Trial Protocol: An intervention to reduce risk factors for childhood obesity in economically and educationally disadvantaged populations. *BMC Public Health, 11*,581. doi:10.1186/1471-2458-11-581 7

Huebner, D. M., Thoma, B. C., & Neilands, T. B. (2015). School victimization and substance use among lesbian, gay, bisexual, and transgender adolescents. *Prevention Science, 16*(5), 734–43. doi:10.1007/s11121-014-0507-x

Human Resources Management Practice.com. https://hrmpractice.com/category/training/. Accessed June, 2019.

Hutchinson, P., Meekers, D., Wheeler, J., Hemblin, J., Anglewicz, P., Silvestre, E., & Keating, J. (2012). External evaluation of the southern African regional social and behavior change communication program, as implemented in Namibia. Tulane University School of Public Health and Tropical Medicine.

Jackson, R. A., Stotland, N. E., Caughey, A. B., & Gerbert, B. (2011). Improving diet and exercise in pregnancy with video doctor counseling: A randomized trial. *Patient Education and Counseling, 83*(2), 203–209, doi:10.1016/j.pec.2010.05.019

Jana, M., Letsela, L., Scheepers, E., & Weiner, R. (2015). Understanding the role of the OneLove campaign in facilitating drivers of social and behavioral change in southern Africa: A qualitative evaluation. *Journal of Health Communication, 20*(3), 252–258. doi:10.1080/1081030.2014.925014

Johnson, S. R. (August 22, 2015). Learning to be LGBT-friendly: Systems train providers to consider sexual, gender orientation in all treatment decisions. *Modern Healthcare.* https://www.modernhealthcare.com/article/20150822/MAGAZINE/308229979

Kelly, M. P., & Barker, M. (2016). Why is changing health-related behaviour so difficult? *Public Health, 136,* 109–16. doi:10.1016/j.puhe.2016.03.030

Kensinger, E. A. (2009) Remembering the details: Effects of emotion. *Emotion Review, 1*(2), 99–113. doi:10.1177/1754073908100432

King James Bible (n.d.). Crossway Bibles. https://www.openbible.info

Kok, G., Peters, L. W. H., Ruiter, R. A. C. (2017). Planning theory and evidence-based behavior change interventions: A conceptual review of the intervention mapping protocol. *Psicologia: Reflexao y Criticia, 30*(1):19. doi:10.1186/s41655-017-0072-x

Kurtovich, E., Ivey, S. L., Neuhauser, L., Graham, C., Constantine, W., & Barkan, H. (2010). Evaluation of a multilingual mass communication intervention for seniors and people with disabilities on Medicaid: A randomized controlled trial. *Health Services Research, 45*(2), 397–417. doi:10.1111/j.1475-6773.2009.01073.x

Lee, Tarryn J., Cameron, Linda D., Wünsche, B., & Stevens, C. (2011). A randomized trial of computer-based communications using imagery and text information to alter representations of heart disease risk and motivate protective behaviour, *British Journal of Health Psychology, 16*(Pt. 1), 72–91. doi:10.1348/135910710X511709

Longman Dictionary. Training. https://www.ldoceonline.com/dictionary/training

Loughrey, M. (2008). Just how male are male nurses? *Journal of Clinical Nursing, 17*(10), 1327–1334. doi:10.1111/j.1365-2702.2007.02250.x

Mayer, K. H., Bradford, J. B., Makadon, H. J., Stall, R., & Goldhammer, H. (2008). Sexual and gender minority health: What we know and what needs to be done. *American Journal of Public Health,* 98L888–995. doi:10.2105/AJPH.2007.127811

McGinty, D. T. (2008). [Review of the book, Serotonin and Sleep: Molecular, Functional, and Clinical Aspects. By J. M. Monti, C. R. Pandi-Perumai, B. L. Jacobs, & D. J. Nutt (Eds.)] *Sleep, 32*(5), 699–700.

Meeusen, R., Watson, P., Hasegawa, H., Roelands, B., & Piacentini, M. F. (2006). Central fatigue: The serotonin hypothesis and beyond. *Sports Medicine, 36*(10), 881–909.

Meis, N., & Kashima, Y. (2017). Signage as a tool for behavioral change: Direct and indirect routes to understanding the meaning of a sign. *PloS One, 12*(8), e0182975. doi:10.1371/journal.pone.0182975

Mirza, S. (2015). Serotonin and depression. *British Medical Journal, 350,* h1771. doi:10.1136/bmj.h1771

Mitchell, K. M., Lee, L., Green, A., & Sykes, J. (2016). The gaps in health care of the LGBT community: Perspectives of nursing students and faculty. Papers & Publications: *Interdisciplinary Journal of Undergraduate Research, 5*(5). https://digitalcommons.northgeorgia.edu/cgi/viewcontent.cgi?article=1178&context=papersandpubs

Movement Enhancement Project (2018). Non-Discrimination Laws. (Updated November 8, 2018). http://www.lgbtmap.org/equality-maps/non_discrimination_laws

Nama, N., MacPherson, P., Sampson, M., & McMillan, H. J. (2017). Medical students' perception of lesbian, gay, bisexual, and transgender (LGBT) discrimination in their learning environment and their self-reported comfort level for caring for LGBT patients: A survey study. *Medical Education Online, 22*(1). doi:10.1080/10872981.2017.1368850

Newport, F. (Dec. 22, 1017). 2017 Update on Americans and Religion, https://news.gallup.com /poll/224642/2017-update-americans-religion.aspx

Nørgaard, M., Ganz, M., Svarer, C., Fisher, P. M., Churchill, N. W., Beliveau, V., ... Knudsen, G. M. (2017). Brain networks implicated in seasonal affective disorder: A neuroimaging PET study of the serotonin transporter. *Frontiers in Neuroscience, 11*, 614. doi:10.3389/fnins .2017.00614

Obedin-Maliver, J., Goldsmith, E. S., Stewart, L., White, W., Tran, E., Brenman, S., ... Lunn, M. R. (2011). Lesbian, gay, bisexual, and transgender-related content in undergraduate medical education. *JAMA, 306*(9), 971–977. doi:10.1001/jama.2011.1255

Oduaran, C. & Nelson, O. Edutainment and HIV/AIDS in Botswana: A content analytical discourse on "Morwalela" drama series. *Online Journal of Communication and Media Technologies, 9*(1), e201901.

Orozco-Olvera, V., Shen, F., & Cluver, L. (2019). The effectiveness of using entertainment education narratives to promote safer sexual behaviors of youth: A meta-analysis, 1985-2017. *PLoS One, 14*(2). doi:10.137/journal.pone.0209969

Out & Equal Workplace Advocates (2018). The 2017 Workplace Equality Fact Sheet, www .outandequal.org/2017-workplace-equality, accessed August 5, 2018.

Oxford English Dictionary. Sexual Orientation. https://www.lexico.com/en/definition/sexual _orientation

Parry, M. (2011). Broadcasting birth control: Family planning and mass media 1914–1984, Dissertation Abstracts International Section A: *Humanities and Social Sciences, 2011, 71*(11-A), 4059, 0419–4209.

Peterson, C. H., Dalley, L. M., Dombrowsi, S. C., & Maier, C. (2017). A review of instruments that measure LGBTQ aftermath and discrimination constructs in adults. *Journal of LGBT Issues in Counseling, 11*(4), 230–246. doi:10.1080/15538605.2017.1380555

Pew Research Center (2019). In U.S., Decline of Christianity Continues at Rapid Pace. An Update on America's Changing Religious Landscape. https://www.pewforum.org/2019/10/17/in-u-s -decline-of-christianity-continues-at-rapid-pace/

Pew Research Center, Gallup Daily Tracking Survey (2016). 5 Key Findings about LGBT by Anna Brown, Factank: News in Numbers, June 13, 2017. https://www.pewresearch.org, accessed June 25, 2019.

Princeton's Word net. Training. http://wordnetweb.princeton.edu/perl/webwn?s=training&sub =Search+WordNet&o2=&o0=1&o8=1&o1=1&o7=&o5=&o9=&o6=&o3=&o4=&h=

Read J. L., & Shortell, S. M. (2011). Interactive games to promote behavior change in prevention and treatment. *JAMA (Online First), 305*(16), 1704–1705. doi:10.1001/jama.2011.408

Risdon, C., Cook, D., & Willms, D. (2000). Gay and lesbian physicians in training: A qualitative study, *Canadian Medical Association Journal, 162*(3), 331–334.

Rocha-Goldberg, M. D. P., Corsino, L., Batch, B., Voils, C. I., Thorpe, C. T., Bosworth, H. B., & Svetkey, L. P. (2010). Hypertension Improvement Project (HIP) Latino: Results of a pilot study of lifestyle intervention for lowering blood pressure in Latino adults. *Ethnicity & Health, 15*(3), 269–282.

Saad, L. (May 15, 2017). Record few Americans believe bible is literal word of God. *Gallup News, Social & Policy Issues*, May 15, 2017 https://news.gallup.com/poll/210704/record-few -americans-believe-bible-literal-word-god.aspx

Schvey, N. A., Blubaugh, J., Morettini, A., & Klein, D. A. (2017). Military family physicians' readiness for treating patients with gender dysphoria. *JAMA Internal Medicine, 177*(5), 727–729.

Schwegman, D. (2018). Rental market discrimination against same-sex couples: Evidence from a pairwise-matched email correspondence test. *Housing Policy Debate, 29*(3), 1–23. doi:10.1080 /10511482.2018.1512005

Sekoni, A. O., Gale, N. K., Manga-Atangana, B., Bhadhuri, A., & Jolly, K. (2017). The effects of educational curricula and training on LGBT-specific health issues for healthcare students and professionals: A mixed-method systematic review. *Journal of the International AIDS Society, 20*(1), 21624. doi:10.7448/IAS.20.1.21624

Shuldman M., & Tajik M. (2010). The role of media/video production in non-media disciplines: The case of health promotion. *Learning, Media and Technology, 35*(3), 357–362

Singh, S., & Durso, L. E. (May 2, 2017). Widespread discrimination continues to shape LGBT people's lives in both subtle and significant ways. *American Progress*, Center for American Progress. https://www.americanprogress.org/issues/lgbt/news/2017/05/02/429529/widespread -discrimination-continues-shape-lgbt-peoples-lives-subtle-significant-ways/

Slater, M. D., & Hayes A. F. (2010). The influence of youth music television viewership on changes in cigarette use and association with smoking peers: A social development, reinforcing spirals perspective. *Communication Research, 37*(6), 751–773.

Substance Abuse and Mental Health Services Administration (SAMHSA) (n.d.). Behavioral health equity. LGBT Training curricula for behavioral health and primary care practitioners. https://www.samhsa.gov/behavioral-health-equity/lgbt/curricula

Surrette, T. E. (2018). Controversial credits: Secondary students' education on heteronormativity. (Doctor of Philosophy Dissertation). University of Calgary, Calgary, Alberta, Canada.

Szymanski, D. M., & Balsam, K. F. Insidious trauma: Examining the relationship between heterosexism and lesbians' PTSD symptoms. *Traumatology, 17*(2), 4–13.

United States Census Bureau, Quick Facts. Population Estimated for July 1, 2018. Accessed May 20, 2019. https://www.census.gov/quickfacts/fact/table/US/PST045218

U.S. Equal Employment Opportunity Commission. (EEOC). *Title VII of the Civil Rights Act of 196*, https://www.eeoc.gov/laws/statutes/titlevii.cfm

Vermeir, E., Jackson, L. A., & Marshall, E. G. (2018). Barriers to primary and emergency care for trans adults. *Culture, Health & Sexuality, 20*(2), 232–246. doi:10.1080/13691058.2017.1338757

Walsh, K. (2005). Edutainment? *British Medical Journal, 330*(7500), 1126.

Wiktionary. Training. https://en.wiktionary.org/wiki/training

Wilson, T. D., & Gilbert, D. T. (2005). Affective forecasting: Knowing what to want. *Current Directions in Psychological Sciences, 14*:3, 131–134. doi:10.1111/j.0963-7214. 2005.00355.x

Wolfensberger, A., Anagnostopoulos, A., Clack, L., Meier, M-T., Kuster, S. P., & Sax, H. (2019). Effectiveness of an edutainment video teaching standard precautions—A randomized controlled evaluation study. *Antimicrobial Resistance & Infection Control, 8*(1), 82. doi:10.1186 /s13756-019-0531-5

Yourdictionary.com. Training. https://www.yourdictionary.com/training

Zeedyk, M. S., & Wallace, L. (2003). Tackling children's road safety through edutainment: An evaluation of effectiveness. *Health Education Research, 18*(4), 493–505.

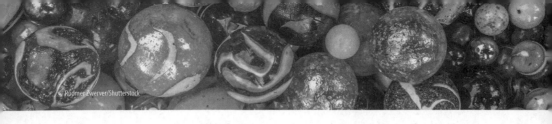

CHAPTER 6

Reducing Isms as Barriers to Output Maximization in Healthcare and Other Workplaces

"I'm the owner of a health care consulting firm and a P.A. by training. Yet, this I know… genetically speaking, all human beings on earth are cousins! Why do we hurt ourselves by treating each other so badly"?

– Jean Drummond, President/CEO HCDI International

LEARNING OBJECTIVES

After completing this chapter, each reader will be able to:

- Review and analyze recent Equal Employment Opportunity Commission (EEOC) cases involving healthcare workplaces.
- List at least two of the EEOC's workplace certification requirements.
- Define and identify implicit bias.
- Define and identify five or more types of nonverbal communications that may generate workplace tensions.
- Analyze recommended strategies that can be used in order to increase output maximization in diverse healthcare and other workplaces.

▶ Introduction: Documented Cases of Isms in Healthcare Workplaces

Isms do exist in American and other healthcare workplaces. These adverse beliefs, attitudes, and behaviors can turn into racism/ethnocentrism, sexism, ageism, lookism, linguicism, anti-semitism, sectarianism, nameism, sizeism, classism, cisgenderism, colorism/shadeism, saneism, and other categories that become associated with incivilities. As mentioned in Chapter 1, Isms operate across numerous groups, and, in the process, create problems that serve as barriers to productivity. Smith (2017) describes key employment cases involving workforce actions that were disruptive to productivity. These cases were based on gender minorities, workers with disabilities, and other subgroups. **BOX 6.1** documents the operation of Isms by listing a sample of relatively recent Equal Employment Opportunity Commission (EEOC) cases in healthcare workplaces.

BOX 6.1 A Sample of EEOC Cases Involving Healthcare Workplaces

- On March 12, 2020, Olympia Senior Care Providers were ordered to settle a **sexual harassment** lawsuit for $450,000.
- On February 20, 2020, Prestige Care and Prestige Senior Living was ordered to pay $2 million to settle an EEOC **disability discrimination** suit.
- On February 11, 2020, the EEOC sued Yale New Haven Hospital on the grounds of age and **disability discrimination**.
- On February 10, 2020, the EEOC sued the White River Health System for **age discrimination**.
- On January 16, 2020, the Medstar Good Samaritan Hospital and EEOC came to an agreement for the sum of $195,000 to settle an EEOC **disability discrimination** suit.
- On July 30, 2019, ChenMed LLC & PMR Virginia Holding LLC was ordered to pay $200,000 in settlement of a **disability discrimination** suit.
- On August 28, 2019, a **sexual harassment** suit culminated in a settlement amount of $200,000 to be paid by A Plus Care Solutions.
- On August 8, 2019, Matrix Medical was ordered to pay $150,000 in settlement of a **pregnancy discrimination** lawsuit.
- On September 11, 2019, Lexington Treatment/Treatment Centers LLC were ordered to pay $110,000 in a **racial harassment** lawsuit.
- On November 21, 2019, a **pregnancy discrimination** case brought against Regency Park Assisted Living.
- On October, 17, 2019, Smiley Dental settled a **pregnancy discrimination** lawsuit.
- On May, 17, 2019, Arizona Health Companies was ordered to pay $545,000 in a Disability and **pregnancy discrimination** case.
- On May 16, 2019, a nationwide **disability discrimination** suit was settled for $950,000 with Corizon Health /Corizon LLC.
- On April 16, 2019, Pulmonary Specialists of Tyler and Sleep Health were ordered to pay $30,000 in settlement for a **disability discrimination**.
- On April 11, 2019, Pruitt Health of Raleigh, North Carolina, settled a lawsuit for $25,000 regarding an EEOC suit based on alleged violations of laws regarding **pregnant women** in workplaces.
- On March 19, 2019, Blue Cross/Blue Shield was told to pay $75,000 in settlement of a **disability discrimination** lawsuit.
- On September 26, 2018, A **sexual harassment and retaliation** suit was filed against Anna's Care.
- On September 25, 2018, Life Care Centers of America was the subject of a **pregnancy discrimination** lawsuit.
- On September 25, 2018, Nix Hospitals System, LLC (dba Nix Healthcare System Services) was for **pregnancy discrimination**.

(continues)

BOX 6.1   A Sample of EEOC Cases Involving Healthcare Workplaces   *(continued)*

- On September 24, 2018, Community Care Health Network was the subject of a **pregnancy discrimination** suit.
- On September 19, 2018, Medstar Washington Hospital Center and Medstar Health was sued for **disability discrimination and retaliation**.
- On September 14, 2018, Happy Valley Nursing and Rehabilitation was sued for **sexual harassment and retaliation**.
- On August 16, 2018, a **religious discrimination** suit was filed against Hackensack Meridian Health.
- On August 9, 2018, a **sexual harassment and retaliation** suit was brought against Amada Senior Care.
- On July 11, 2018, a **disability discrimination** suit was brought up against Dignity Health.
- On July 6, 2018, TrueCore Behavioral Solutions was ordered to pay $38,000 in settlement of an **Equal Pay and Title VII** lawsuit.
- On June 28, 2018, a suit was filed against Hawaii Medical Service Association for **Class disability discrimination**.
- On May 30, 2018, St. Vincent Hospital in Indianapolis, Indiana, was ordered to pay $15,000 in settlement of a **disability discrimination** lawsuit.
- On May 15, 2018, Foothill Child Development Center of Upland, California, also settled an EEOC **disability discrimination** case.
- On May 11, 2018, SCION Dental whose parent company is SKYGEN, was referred to trial for a case involving **racial/ethnic acts** that occurred in the workplace.
- On May 2, 2018, the Children's Home of Tampa, Florida, settled a lawsuit based upon **gender-based treatment issues** in their workplace.
- On April 26, 2018, a group of workers were awarded $5.1 million regarding four alleged **religion-based workplace violations** for select workers employed by the United Health Program of America Incorporated and Costs Containment Group Incorporated.
- On March 7, 2018, a legal suit was brought by the EEOC against Scottish Pines Rehabilitation and Nursing Center in Charlotte, North Carolina, for **pregnancy discrimination**.
- On February 4, 2018, a case was brought against Memorial Health Care of Detroit, Michigan, for **religious discrimination**.
- On January 12, 2018, the Mission Hospital of Asheville, North Carolina, signed paperwork to pay $89,000 based on a **religious discrimination** case.
- On January 10, 2018, Pioneer Health Services of Jacksonville, Mississippi settled a **disability discrimination** suit for $85,000.
- On January 4, 2018, Montrose Memorial Hospital of Montrose, Colorado settled an **age discrimination** lawsuit for $400,000.
- On December 22, 2017, Dependable Health Services in Baltimore, Maryland, was ordered to pay $38,000 as a settlement in a **disability discrimination** suit.
- On December 20, 2017, Trinity Hospital in Minneapolis, Minnesota, was required to pay $95,000 as part of a **pregnancy discrimination** lawsuit.
- On December 1, 2017, Accent Care of Dallas, Texas, was requested to pay $25,000 as part of a **disability discrimination** case.
- On November 13, 2017, Community Pharmacy in San Diego, California, settled an **unequal pay discrimination** case for $60,000.
- On November 1, 2017, Phoebe Putney Hospital in Atlanta Georgia was sued by the EEOC in a **disability discrimination** case.

- On October 25, 2017, Professional Endodontics in Detroit, Michigan, was sued for **age discrimination**.
- On October 3, 2017, The Children's Home, Inc. of Tampa, Florida, was sued by the EEOC for **sex discrimination** and retaliation.
- On September 29, 2017, Prestige Senior Living of Fresno, California, was sued by the EEOC for **disability discrimination**.
- On September 25, 2017, Trinity Health of Livonia, Michigan, was sued for **pregnancy discrimination**.
- On September 25, 2017, Georgia Blue Cross was sued for withdrawing a job offer to a newly hired employee who required **religious accommodations**.
- On September 20, 2017, Louisville Medical Practice in Louisville, Kentucky, was sued on the basis of **religious discrimination and retaliation**.
- On August 14, 2017, Dependable Health Services of Baltimore, Maryland, was sued for **disability discrimination**.
- On July 25, 2017, Home Instead, Alameda In-Home Senior Care provider of San Francisco, California, was sued for **sex and race harassment and for retaliation**.

Data from United States Equal Employment Opportunity Commission. (EEOC) Selected Case Lists. https://www.eeoc.gov/eeoc /litigation/selected/index.cfm

As the described cases suggest, despite the use of in-person and/or online training, healthcare workplaces are represented among those industries and employers who, for various reasons, are noncompliant with the current laws that are monitored by the EEOC. In 2019, the EEOC (2020) reports that there were 23,532 filings (32.4% of all 2019 charges) for sex-based discrimination activities which included 12,739 sexual harassment charges (EEOC Charge Statistics National FY (1997–2019)). Moreover, there were 23,976 (33.0%) cases revolving around racial issues, and 2,725 cases (3.7%) based on religious discrimination. Many of these were in the healthcare industry. As the data suggest, various Isms exist in healthcare workplaces. While the specific "Isms" included in the EEOC data do not cover everything, the cases listed confirm the need for healthcare administrators, managers, and human resources managers to collectively seek to implement interventions that reverse the operation of such forces in their health-care organizations.

▶ Reducing Isms in Healthcare Workplaces: Strategy #1: The Role of the EEOC

It would be impossible to discuss Isms in healthcare and/or other workplaces without out a detailed discussion of the U.S. Equal Employment Opportunity Commission (EEOC). As is known, the **EEOC** is an external support system for healthcare and other workplaces whose workers experience negative behavior based on various "Isms." However, EEOC solutions do not constitute a productivity strategy for any workplace. Indeed, by the time such beliefs, attitudes, and behaviors are transformed into EEOC cases, productivity has already decreased. Nevertheless, it is important for healthcare managers and human resources managers to be familiar with how the EEOC operates. This is because the management of EEOC cases is a part of their responsibility. Whether evaluating compliance to the findings in Garcia, Buitrago, United Food and Commercial Workers, AFL-CIO versus Spun Steak, or investigating cases involving whistle-blowing in healthcare workplaces based upon precedences established by Hopkins vs. City of Midland, the United States EEOC is mandated to identify and respond to the intrusion of adverse personal and/or institutional incivilities associated with isms that occur in America's labor markets. Initially established under the auspices of Title IV of the 1964 Civil Rights Act, numerous laws, executive orders, and/or judicial decisions provide the operational framework used by the EEOC in monitoring, reviewing, and responding to claims of unbalanced treatment involving recruitment, hiring, training, compensation, evaluation, planning, discipline, termination, and all other areas of human resources management.

The processes involved in serving as the nation's federal agency for the protection of those who would otherwise be emotionally and mentally disenfranchised through direct and/or indirect acts of asymmetric treatment are highly sensitive. Healthcare administrators and managers are aware that the EEOC is legally required to protect those who have been treated unfairly. Yet, the agency must not violate the rights of healthcare and other workplaces that have been unfairly accused. The EEOC is required to act promptly and fairly in recommending remediation for those who have been made "victims" through behavioral and/or systemic forces. The EEOC's management of its complex workload underlies the need for quick and accurate systems for the management of more than 290,000 pieces of mail annually; a variable quantity of printing; the duplication of more than 1,900,000 copies of various documents; the movement and transportation of furniture and supplies; the management of, access to, safety of, and the cleanliness of the EEOC's various physical facilities; the filing, storage, retrieval, transport, and destruction of records; the management of space; the writing and updating of directives, and a number of other services to EEOC sites located throughout the country. The excellent and accurate delivery of services allows the United States EEOC to confidently and efficaciously complete the very serious management duties that it is legislated to perform—the approval of the filing of civil rights discrimination cases under current legislation.

It is also necessary to remind healthcare administrators and managers that the EEOC's primary duty is not to bring cases. Rather, the agency actively seeks to *prevent* activities that result in cases. One approach is requiring all workplaces to have EEOC certification. The EEOC certification is based on agreements by all employers, contractors, vendors, and suppliers that each individual employed by the organization and/or its affiliates or business partners receive fair treatment that does not differ because of race/ethnicity, sex, ancestry, national origin, disability status, pregnancy status, nor other characteristics that are not directly related to the workers' ability to complete the duties outlined in their job descriptions. To support this outcome, the EEOC certification process for employers and/or contractors requires each component listed in **BOX 6.2**.

Moreover, when healthcare workplaces are the subject of inquiry, this agency understands how healthcare workplaces operate. Indeed, EEOC materials can be adapted by workplaces to reduce the growth of Isms. For example, the U.S. EEOC, Office of Federal Operations fully understands the multi-layered complexity of healthcare and other workplaces. Accordingly, the EEOC itself offers a range of

BOX 6.2　Basic Requirements for a Workplace to Be EEOC Compliant		
The employer or contractor has a written policy statement prohibiting discrimination in all phases of employment.	☐ Yes	☐ No
The employer or contractor periodically conducts his or her own self-analysis or utilization analysis of the workforce.	☐ Yes	☐ No
The employer or contractor has a system for determining if its employment practices are discriminatory against protected people.	☐ Yes	☐ No
The employer or contractor, when problem areas are identified in employment practices, has a system for taking reasonable corrective action. This policy must, however, include the establishment of goals or timetables for resolution.	☐ Yes	☐ No

EEOC. https://www.eeoc.gov/employers/eeo1survey/faq.cfm#TypesOReports

courses that, while primarily directed toward people employed by the federal government, can also be used as a training model in healthcare and other workplaces. **BOX 6.3** lists a few courses that the U.S. EEOC has offered recently.

Courses such as those listed can be introduced into healthcare workplaces as preventive training programs for existing employees. These courses can also be used by human resources managers to alert new and current workers about EEOC's most recent laws and the court's interpretation of these laws. Of course, such courses are not directly available to all workers in healthcare and other workplaces. Rather, the amount of detail that would be covered if a healthcare workplace decided to mimic this approach from the EEOC is such that the training would primarily be for people in management who are choosing to serve as the equivalent of an EEOC counselor, attorney, program coordinator, and/or as a Diversity Investigator/EEO Investigator for that particular healthcare organization. Thus, by creating these countermeasures, healthcare workplaces can prevent circumstances

BOX 6.3　A Sample of EEOC Courses That Can Be Modified for Use in Healthcare and/or Other Places
■ Anti-Harassment Program Management ■ Disability Basics ■ Barrier Analysis ■ EEO Laws Refresher ■ EEO Training for Counselors and Investigators

Constructed by the Authors based upon EEOC research. EEOC Training Institute https://eeotraining.eeoc.gov/

that lead to the type of previously described EEOC healthcare cases. Similarly, the EEOC seeks to keep organizations educated. This is because the EEOC cannot hold organizations that fall within its regulatory scope accountable for adherence to its agenda without a system for communicating and educating the public regarding past, current, new, and proposed regulations or rulings. Using the EEOC model, human resources managers in healthcare workplaces must keep both managers and workers up-to-date regarding changing laws and policies. As is true for the EEOC, the HR department must develop and distribute compliance manuals that describe, in simple language, the implications of legislative, judicial, and executive mandates upon the human resources decisions of their organizations. Additionally, the EEOC's accomplishment of its annual goals require that its standards, preferred practices, protocols, and operational guidelines be shared with its employees and contractual staff.

In order to achieve these goals, the EEOC operates a Directive System. It is important that the healthcare organization's HR Department have its own version of a Directive System. As is true for EEOC, the organization's healthcare Directive System will complete tasks such as researching and tracking EEOC policy changes and/or alterations by gathering memoranda, meeting minutes, and other written materials regarding a regulation or programmatic issue. While the EEOC assigns a team of writers that consists of labor law experts, labor experts, labor economists, and wage specialists to provide the services, the HR division can assign staff to perform the same functions. The initial step for the staff should be to search regulations.gov for EEOC documents. The staff should also search the Federal Register, Title 29 of the Code of Federal Regulations (CFR), and hold meetings with Administrators and Managers and the General Counsel of the healthcare organization. The internal team can also use different methods and materials to obtain all of EEOC's current and past directives. These directives are separated into **external directives** and **internal directives**.

The EEOC's staff separates materials into external directives that are assigned to the labor attorney and the labor economist for review and analysis. The internal directives are assigned to HR Specialists. Each team then reviews and catalogs the directives by type. For example, *external directives* are identified. These include materials such as the EEOC's Guidelines on Discrimination Because of Sex, Guidelines on Discrimination Because of Religion, and other directives that introduce the criteria used by the EEOC to define alternative types of discrimination. Similarly, **investigational directives** are grouped together. These include documents such as *Procedures for Coordinating the Investigation of Complaints or Charges of Employment Discrimination* based *on Disability Subject to the Americans with Disabilities Act and Sector 504 of the Rehabilitation Act of 1973*, and related directives that guide the collection of evidence to support an EEOC claim. While this precise process cannot be duplicated by all healthcare organizations, parallel procedures should certainly be followed by HR staff in larger healthcare workplaces.

At a minimum, in larger healthcare organizations, the total of EEOC's internal and external directives should be reviewed, classified, and grouped on an annual basis. Each large HR department should also conduct a literature review and gather published articles from journals and government publications that relate to each directive. These materials can be arranged from the most recent to the oldest. Each

---

BOX 6.4 How to Use an Internal Directive

HR must ask:

- Does our healthcare workplace adhere to each directive?
- Do our directives reflect state-of-the-art knowledge regarding all programmatic issues?
- Does someone on our staff have the level of literacy that is needed to understand the information in the directive?
- To what degree does the literacy level of the directive match that of the intended audience?
- What changes would users of external and/or internal directives like to see in the document?

---

directive should be analyzed within the context of other directives and related literature. A summary can be created that analyzes each of the directives. Recommendations can then be made to improve adherence to these materials. Those recommendations should be discussed with a team including all managers. The recommendations made can then be put into a written report. **BOX 6.4** lists some of the areas that the HR Department should address.

Based on the above questions and methods, the workplace's team can then make evidence-based recommendations regarding adherence to directives. The EEOC Directives System ensures that directives that the EEOC selects for reissuance are written in simple, non-legal language. For example, the EEOC Compliance Manual is an excellent example of the use of a Plain Language Format. The healthcare workplace's HR Department must ensure that all of their materials are easy to understand.

This federal agency ensures that healthcare and other workplaces have the information required to prevent cases from being brought before the EEOC. Healthcare administrators and managers cannot prevent Isms in their workplace without knowledge of similar prevention strategies that are or could be relevant to their workplaces.

In other words, healthcare institutions will benefit by similarly tracking all EEOC activities that involve the healthcare industry and by institutionalizing similar practices. Fewer legal cases will be brought against healthcare institutions if such approaches are applied.

▶ Reducing Isms in Healthcare Workplaces: Stategy #2: The Critical Role of the Analysis of the Risk of "Isms"

As the analysis of selected adverse beliefs, attitudes, and behaviors in healthcare and other workplaces has shown, many of the highly critical barriers to high workplace productivity have not yet been identified. Accordingly, the development of more effective strategies to reducing the existence of Isms in healthcare workplaces requires that healthcare administrators, managers, and human resources staff examine the concept of discrimination more deeply. This is because the concept of discrimination has become so frequently used that it often oversimplifies this very complex phenomenon. In an effort to better understand workplace relationships, Lepak and Snell (1999) describe all workplaces as having a "human resource architecture." They also said that workplace problems will emerge because in any given workplace, there will be a differential distribution of the ownership and operationalization of "…the knowledge and skills that are of strategic importance (page 31)."

This is an important first step to understanding the tensions and conflicts that can emerge in diverse healthcare and other workplaces because of central tendency. As a result of central tendencyism, some subgroups of employees assume that the "ownership of knowledge and skills that are of strategic importance" to the workplace outcomes are differentially distributed across subgroups. Thus, in healthcare workplaces, some patients view subgroups as not being equal in the "…knowledge and skills that are of equal importance."

Evidence suggests that negative opinions exist regarding the relationship between diverse workplaces and productivity. **BOX 6.5** introduces some supporting evidence that some persons believe that workplaces characterized by varied human differences reduce rather than enhance productivity.

If a person were to analyze such positions, it becomes clear that the resistance to diverse workforces may be based on the belief that culturally diverse populations under-perform in the workplace and, as a result, do not support the maximization of output. Yet, there is considerable evidence that confirms that culturally diverse groups and subgroups do not reduce productivity in workplaces. For example, economists recognize that, to some degree, the income earned by workers reflects their marginal productivity. Thus, to some degree, income is a measure of workplace success. **TABLE 6.1** describes a ranking of the median household income for a number of America's ethnic-based groups. These data may surprise many employees and employers.

As Table 6.1 reveals, diverse groups in American society obviously make tremendous contributions to productivity in order to generate this sample distribution of earnings. Additionally, Richard et al. (2000) conducted an analysis of workplace productivity, the financial return on equity, and overall marketplace outcomes.

BOX 6.5 "Evidence" That Some Workers Believe That Culturally Diverse Workers and Workplaces Reduce Rather Than Enhance Output Maximization

- Allen et al. (2007), in a study of 391 managers and 130 organizations in the southeastern United States, found that these managers and professionals believed that organizational performance was inversely proportional to the degree of cultural diversity in upper management. In other words, it was believed that the more diverse upper management was, the less productive the workplace was.
- In a study of various measures to increase the equitable operation of diverse workplaces, Dobbin et al. (2015) concluded that "…some popular bureaucratic reforms thought to quell discrimination, instead activated it" (page 32). The notion that "diversity is the path to political and cultural extinction is a view held by some persons in the American workforce."

TABLE 6.1 Ranking of Household Income of America's Ethnic-Based Group			
1. Indian Americans	$107,390[1]	9. Greek-Americans	$77,342[1]
2. Jewish Americans	$97,500[2]	10. Lebanese Americans	$74,757[1]
3. Taiwanese Americans	$85,566[3]	11. Sri Lankan Americans	$73,856[1]
4. Filipino Americans	$82,389[3]	12. Croatian Americans	$73,196[1]
5. Australian Americans	$81,452[1]	13. Latvian Americans	$72,690[1]
6. Israeli Americans	$79,736[1]	14. Lithuanian Americans	$72,605[1]
7. European Americans	$77,440[1]	15. Austrian Americans	$72,478[1]
8. Russian Americans	$77,349[1]		

Data from : 1) "Median household income in the past 12 months (and 2015 inflation-adjusted dollars)." American Community Survey. United States Census Bureau. 2015. Retrieved 3 December 2016; 2) Amy Chua, Jed Rubenfeld (2014). The Triple Package How Three Unlikely Traits Explain the Rise and Fall of Cultural Groups in America. Penguin Press HC. P. 53. ISBN 978-159425460; 3) "Median household income in the past 12 months (and 2014 inflation-adjusted dollars)." American Community Survey. United States Census Bureau. 2014. Retrieved 3 December 2015.

They found that more culturally diverse companies outperformed those who were not from as diverse a background. Based on data from the 1996 to 1997 National Organizations Survey, Herring (2009) also found that racial/ethnic diversity was correlated with higher revenues, a larger customer base, and higher profits. Eagly (2016), however, emphasizes that diversity can have no effect and/or a negative effect on productivity and urges researchers to be totally honest when trying to find the answer to this question.

This finding suggests that additional research is needed to identify conditions under which culturally diverse workplaces can achieve higher productivity. For example, Desai et al. (2014), conducted five studies based upon 993 heterosexually married males and identified a set of dynamics that operate in contemporary workplaces regarding women. Specifically, these authors discovered that when workplaces include married males whose wives were not in the labor market, a number of barriers to high productivity became a reality. First, the males were more likely to be biased toward the women in these workplaces. Second, these males were more likely to subjectively perceive the workplaces' operations to be less efficient. Third, the males in the samples were resistant to workplaces in which females were in managerial and/or administrative positions. Fourth, when placed in a position to do so, such males were more likely to behave in a discriminatory fashion toward females when it came to financial and career advancement. Fifth, males who were not married initially but subsequently married women who were not in the labor market, adopted similar attitudes even if they did not feel that way when they were unmarried. This suggests that males and females may both require "education" regarding research findings on the contributions of diverse populations in workplaces so that diversity-related, productivity-inhibiting behaviors can be minimized. Hoobler et al. (2016) analyzed data on 117,639 people in 78 different workplaces. This specific research was to identify the association between female CEOs, top-level managers, and Board of Director members and high productivity as measured by financial performance. The authors concluded that a positive association exists between females' **unconstrained inclusion** and financial outcomes.

The research indicates that cultural diversity can positively and/or negatively impact workplace productivity. When diversity is associated with conflict, output is not maximized. But, as the data reveal, cultural conflict does exist in some healthcare and non-healthcare workplaces. Martin (2014) argues that cultural conflict is often recreated in the workplace through a number of processes including:

- Miscommunication;
- Differences in beliefs and norms that generate a range of nonhomogeneous behaviors that consequently create reactions to these behaviors;
- Historical relationships that result in current day responses;
- Other variables that serve as sources of differences of opinion, reactive behaviors; and conflict.

Factors such as these comprise "constrained inclusion" rather than unconstrained inclusion. Since many workplaces consist of humans who behave negatively based on their adverse beliefs, attitudes, and behaviors, "constrained inclusion" often exists. Thus, the task of healthcare administrators and managers is to identify consultants and researchers who can assist the HR Department in bringing about behavioral changes. The merit of better understanding why certain mechanisms support and maintain "Isms" in the workplaces cannot be overemphasized.

Diversity in healthcare workplaces can, however, also bring about higher productivity. Consider a piano. Because each key on a piano produces a different sound, the outcome can be discordant if a person does not know how to play the piano. However, the different notes and chords can also be magical if the person playing the piano knows how to move the keys harmonically. Likewise, the diversity of nature includes more than 400,000 species of flowers and plants (Edwards, 2010). Multiple combinations and permutations of beautiful flower arrangements can be created that are extraordinary. Healthcare workplaces that reduce the impact of Isms and maximize high productivity can produce a similar outcome. However, higher productivity requires that the potential or actual causes of the ism be analyzed. For example, diverse healthcare workplaces, like workplaces in general, have not yet identified the full range of disparities that may be operative under the surface. This is because the focus of workplace disparities that may impede maximum productivity across America primarily focuses on EEOC violations. The Department of Labor regulates workplaces via the administration and enforcement of more than 180 federal laws. Even under the surface, the range of permutations and combinations of Isms that threaten productivity is numerous. This suggests that each healthcare workplace must self-evaluate at a micro-level. To do so, they must determine why their specific work environments have such an imbalance. Additionally, the audit would seek to answer questions such as those in **BOX 6.6**.

It appears that current healthcare workplaces do not collect and analyze the data described. This conclusion is based on a thorough review of the literature,

BOX 6.6 Who Are We Really? Identifying Structural Disparities in Diverse Healthcare Workplaces—A Micro-Analysis

1. Are there subgroup disparities in the mean number of hours that employees with the same or similar job descriptions worked annually?

   Yes_____ No_____

   If so, are the differences statistically significant?

   Yes_____ No_____

2. Are there subgroup differences in the wages and salaries paid to employees with comparable years of experience, comparable educational backgrounds and, extremely importantly, comparable performance appraisals?

   Yes_____ No_____

   If so, are the differences statistically significant?

   Yes_____ No_____

3. Are there statistically significant subgroup differences in workers' compensation paid by the healthcare organization over each work year?

   Yes_____ No_____

4. Are there statistically significant differences in employee benefits for workers with comparable credentials, work histories, and position descriptions?

   Yes_____ No_____

5. Are there statistically significant differentials in actions taken in terms of employee protections of any type by subgroups even if these employees differ in terms of work tenure, education, position description, years of experience, and/or other factors?

   Yes_____ No_____

6. Are there unexplained statistically significant subgroup differences in the percentage of veterans and/or ex-veterans hired or rejected under the Uniform Services Employment and Re-employment Rights Act?

   Yes_____ No_____

7. Have any differential Employee Polygraph Protection Act violations occurred within your healthcare workplace?

   Yes_____ No_____

8. Are there unexplained statistically significant subgroup differences when handling wage garnishments?

   Yes_____ No_____

9. Are there unexplained statistically significant subgroup differences in hiring under the Veterans Preference measures?

   Yes_____ No_____

10. Are there unexplained statistically significant subgroup differences when awarding government contracts, grants, and/or financial assistance for educational purposes?

    Yes_____ No_____

11. Have unexplained statistically significant differential rates of injuries and accidents occurred among workers holding the same job descriptions and within the same occupations over the last 5 years by subgroups?

    Yes_____ No_____

(continues)

BOX 6.6   Who Are We Really? Identifying Structural Disparities in Diverse
Healthcare Workplaces—A Micro-Analysis   *(continued)*

12. Have unexplained statistically significant differential layoffs or firings occurred
     by subgroup within your healthcare workplace for individuals with the same job
     descriptions?

     Yes_____ No_____

13. Have unexplained statistically significant differentials occurred by subgroup in
     family and medical leave?

     Yes_____ No_____

14. Have unexplained statistically significant similar subgroups been utilized in new
     construction or renovations of your healthcare workplace?

     Yes_____ No_____

15. Are there undercurrents of discord and dissatisfaction in your workplace? If so, do
     these differ by subgroup?

which revealed that no research has been conducted on healthcare workplaces based
upon the described queries. Yet, in the data-oriented environment of contemporary
healthcare workplaces, the HR Department should not only routinely collect such
data but the data should also be analyzed at least once a year so that improvements
in workplace equity can be tracked.

However, healthcare workplaces not only require an overview of their current
diversity practices, it is also necessary to know the **Diversity Dimensions** of the
workplace. For example, as a professional gardener, the person should know the
name, quantity, and origin of all flowers, trees, and other components of the gardens
which they oversee. Accordingly, every HR Department should know exactly how
much diversity exists in the organization. In order to assess the Diversity Dimensions of the healthcare or other organization, a statistical profile of the employees
must be assembled based on demographics, sociographics, and psychographics. Second, once the various nationalities, racial/ethnic groups, age groups, etc., have been
identified, the organization should conduct an analysis that allows intersectional
groups to be identified. This requires analyzing the data to determine the number
and percentage of workers who fit into multiple diverse groups. Third, directly or
through a contractor, implement the psychographic component of the research to
define unique values, beliefs, and behaviors about or toward other subgroups that
these various groups have brought into the healthcare workplace. Based on these
variables, a Diversity Dimensions score can be calculated that measures the risks
of higher productivity being affected by workplace Isms. (A workplace with fewer
intersectionalities will have a lower Diversity Dimensions score than one with many
intersectionalities.)

This recommendation is based on findings from Hardcastle and Hagger (2015).
These researchers argue that although there have been advances in interventions
that increase individuals' engagement in health-related behaviors, there is still a
relative dearth of evidence regarding the processes by which interventions affect
behavior. Later in the article, these analysts emphasize why implementing research
that moves beyond demographic and sociographic profiles only is critical. In order

to bring about a behavioral change, a person must understand the beliefs, attitudes, values, aesthetics, and other aspects of psychographics. Indeed, these analysts imply that whether in the United States, Great Britain, or in any other geographic area where multiple populations exist, major behavioral change will not occur without a more holistic approach. A Diversity Dimensions score is a more holistic approach. Stated differently, Hardcastle and Hagger's work implies that the same strategies that are applied by managerial marketers can be used to induce healthcare behavioral changes. That is, intensive research must be completed and the relevant marketing segments must be identified. These segments must then be further researched and baselined by the philosophical, social, psychological, and other attributes so that newly defined target audiences can be identified for behavioral interventions to be marketed. The information provided by the Diversity Dimensions score will allow the HR Division and other managers to progress beyond EEOC compliance and cultural competency training as tools to generate the behavioral changes needed to increase output maximization.

EEOC compliance and cultural competency training are definitely necessary tools for use in diverse healthcare and other workplaces. Jernigan et al. (2016) cite findings from 18 cultural competency programs that have been used to train physicians in the United States. The results from the evaluation data revealed that in many cases, the "knowledge, attitudes, and skills (page 166)" of the participants improved. However, the unhealthy, dysfunctional behaviors as evidenced by overweight and/or obesity in the healthcare workplace confirms the difficulty that humans encounter in transitioning *from knowledge to behavioral change*. Thus, the Diversity Dimensions score allows EEOC compliance and cultural competency approaches to be supplemented by more comprehensive behavioral change interventions. The need for complementary tools is confirmed by the data in **TABLE 6.2**, which includes data on the total number of EEOC charges filed in the 12-year period from 2007–2019.

As Table 6.2 reveals, a total of 1,167,492 total EEOC charges were filed between 2007 and 2019. These charges were particularly skewed toward race and national origin combined. Sex, age, and disability were other areas that were associated with workplace conflict. Retaliation was also prevalent. Yet, the number of cases per year remained relatively consistent. Such data suggest that current approaches to culturally diverse workplaces require additional strategies. Specifically, interventions are needed in order to bring about *behavioral change* in healthcare and other workplaces. The authors recommend that two highly critical steps be used as starting points.

Step #1: Assess Implicit Bias in Your Healthcare Workplace

As mentioned, annual online, anonymous surveys are needed to collect information on each worker. These surveys can collect key information on demographic, sociographic, and psychographic data. Each worker should be able to anonymously test themselves for hidden bias by using one or more Implicit Bias Association Tests (http://www.tolerance.org). Once analyzed, these data provide a baseline for measuring the change that takes place in the performance appraisal data as changes occur in mean hidden bias scores in the workplace.

TABLE 6.2 EEOC Charges Filed for 2007–2017 All Workplaces by Category

Category↓ # of Charges →	2007	2008	2009	2010	2011	2012	2013	2014	2015	2016	2017	2018	2019
	82,792	95,402	93,277	99,922	99,947	99,412	93,727	88,778	89,385	91,503	84,254	76,418	72,675
■ Race	37.0%	35.6%	36.0%	35.9%	35.4%	33.7%	35.3%	35.0%	34.7%	35.3%	33.9%	32.2%	33.0%
■ Sex	30.1%	29.7%	30.0%	29.1%	28.5%	30.5%	29.5%	29.3%	19.5%	29.4%	30.4%	32.3%	32.4%
■ National Origin	11.4%	11.1%	11.9%	11.3%	11.8%	10.9%	11.4%	10.8%	10.9%	10.8%	9.8%	9.3%	9.6%
■ Religion	3.5%	3.4%	3.6%	3.6%	4.2%	3.8%	4.0%	4.0%	3.9%	4.2%	4.1%	3.7%	3.7%
■ Color	2.1%	2.8%	3.2%	2.8%	2.8%	2.7%	3.4%	3.1%	3.2%	3.4%	3.8%	4.1%	4.7%
■ Retaliation (All statutes)	32.3%	34.3%	36.0%	36.3%	37.4%	38.1%	41.1%	42.8%	44.9%	45.0%	48.8%	51.6%	53.8%
■ Retaliation (Title VII Only)	28.3%	30.1%	30.1%	30.1%	31.4%	31.4%	33.6%	34.7%	35.7%	36.5%	38.0%	40.0%	41.4%
■ Age	23.2%	25.8%	24.4%	23.3%	23.5%	23.5%	23.5%	22.8%	23.2%	21.8%	21.8%	22.1%	21.4%
■ Disability	21.4%	20.4%	23.0%	25.2%	25.8%	26.5%	26.5%	28.2%	30.2%	30.2%	31.9%	32.2%	33.4%
■ Equal Pay	1.0%	1.0%	1.0%	1.0%	0.9%	1.1%	1.1%	1.1%	1.1%	1.2%	1.2%	1.4%	1.5%

Charge Statistics (National FY 1997–2017), U.S. Equal Employment Opportunity Commission, Retrieved from https://www.eeoc.gov/eeoc/statistics/enforcement/charges.cfm

¹Total Charges = 1,167,492 from 2007 to 2019.

Step #2: Implement Training in the Workplace that Contexts the Need for Behavioral Change

Catalyst (2016) advances the argument that it is important to hold discussions regarding gender and race/ethnicity in the workplace. Banks (2016) argues that such discussions are highly critical. Kedem (2016) emphasizes the criticality of holding such discussions in the workplace. Goldbach (2017) provides a toolkit to support workplaces in discussing diversity issues. Other analysts make similar arguments. However, the proposal is that these current approaches be replaced by training that will support a commitment to human life preservation by each worker.

Pamela Arnold (2011) cites a quote from a book by Harris Sussman, *The Future of Diversity and the Work Ahead of Us*. This quote asserts that diversity is literally a paradigm that is used for viewing all that exists. This suggests that it is not diversity in healthcare and other workplaces that generate problems. Rather, it is how diversity is viewed and responded to by various humans. Differences now serve as a source of conflict because the role of human differences in the survival of humankind has been insufficiently integrated into diversity dialogue. Yet, the central question that supports humankind is, "How can we utilize the knowledge, skills, creativity, and other resources of all workers so that output is maximized and the current and future survival of humankind is supported"? Thus, humankind's survival becomes the macro-level context that must support discourse on human differences.

Such a question flows from the domain of philosophy with a particular focus on logic. The Stanford Encyclopedia of Philosophy (n.d.) makes a highly critical differentiation between logic and information. *Logic* is defined in this publication as a *consequence*. In logic, one is reminded that logic is based on "if then" arguments. That is, if the premise X is true, then Y would be the outcome. This differentiation says that training is needed in workplaces in order to reframe employees' thinking so that the focus is on the survival of humankind.

In contrast, *information* is defined as a "commodity." This suggests that the *premise* leads to the consequence. Such a relationship is particularly obvious in healthcare because symptoms of disease/illness (information) are used to correctly diagnose disease/illness (information). This information is then used to select and apply a treatment for the disease/illness (information), which then determines the patient's subsequent mortality and/or morbidity status (outcome). Because the "historic" informational chain is "short" in healthcare, no disconnect occurs in the logical chain between "information" and "consequence."

However, the information that connects humankind to survival is complex. As a consequence, in the contemporary world, information and consequences are easy to analyze incorrectly. All human action has a positive and/or negative impact on the probability of the survival of humankind. Music provides an excellent example.

Schäfer (2016), for example, argues that not only does music serve a function in human lives in terms of emotional regulation, social relationships, etc., but that individuals can increase their chance of survival by choosing the frequency and type of music to which they are exposed. In contrast, Rentfrow (2012), Deutsch (2008)[,] and others introduce evidence that music has a positive impact upon health outcomes. MacDonald (2013) provides a literature review of the impact of music on the health of humankind.

Similarly, humans who work as gardeners ultimately support the survival of mankind. Soga (2017) completed a meta-analysis of empirical studies on the relationship between gardens and health outcomes. The results revealed that a decrease in depression and anxiety accompanies gardening. Even positive body mass index changes were associated with gardening.

Clearly, research supports the overall survival of humankind via the goods and services produced. However, the noted economist, Lester C. Thurow (1978), addressed the legitimacy of the concept of psychic income as a value that would, can, and will, under the correct circumstances, deliver human satisfaction. Thus, benefits that support humankind extend far beyond economic outcomes. Indeed, other researchers have highlighted the range of motivations and activities that contribute to the individual and collective survival of humankind. Healthcare marketplaces become an ideal environment for training that educates individuals regarding behaviors and actions that serve the individual and the collective good. Research such as this supports the thesis that humans engaged in positive output-producing activities support the survival of humankind.

For example, sociologists generally classify human interactions as being based on competition and conflict and/or cooperation and accommodation. Cooperation and accommodation are human interactions that support output maximization within a diverse healthcare and/or other workplace. A hospital, nursing home, medical practice, pharmacy, dialysis center, and/or other healthcare environment produces more positive outcomes when workers see themselves in different roles while serving as *parts of the same team*. However, preliminary research has also determined that people who are on the same team do not compete with each other. For example, Wagner et al. (2002) conducted research on competition that included two teams from the Commonwealth of Dominica. When a team from the same village competed among themselves, their biological readings included lower levels of hormonal changes (i.e., cortisol and testosterone) than when they competed against team members from a different village. More recently, McHale et al. (2018) completed a very interesting article that suggests that individuals who view themselves as a team do not generate the hormonal changes associated with competition when they play against each other in a sports game. However, when these same individuals play against a group whom they view as a different team, increases in hormonal responses occur. Specifically, investigators studied 102 boys in soccer, whose team defined themselves as Chinese and lived in Hong Kong. When the boys played against their own teammates during intra-team matches, no additional testosterone, dehydroepiandrosterone (**DHEA**), androstenedione, or **cortisol** was released. However, when these young males played against soccer players whom they considered to be on a different team, significant ($p < 0.05$) increases occurred in the levels of their health hormones.

Clinical research in health care defines *testosterone* as the steroid hormone primarily produced in the testes of males. *Cortisol* is a stress hormone that is produced in the adrenal glands. Cortisol is associated with crisis. However, the less well-known *dehydroepiandrosterone* (DHEA) is a naturally produced steroid hormone that is produced in the brain, the adrenal glands, and the sexual organs. In contrast, *androstenedione* is also a steroid hormone that is associated with the adrenal glands that is also active in the production of testosterone. McHale et al.'s research, when extrapolated to diversity issues, reveals that "Isms" in the workplace cause people who are different to see each other as "…not a part of the same team."

Viewing one's colleagues in a healthcare or other workplace as members of a "different team" can generate higher levels of hormones. These higher levels of hormones have been found to be associated with more aggression in some studies. Carrè et al. (2017) found that such an outcome primarily occurs among males that have a high dominance score and a low self-control rating. Prasad et al. (2017) completed research that determined that the existence of a relationship between levels of male hormones and the emergence of retaliatory behavior. Accordingly, whether people who work in healthcare and other workplaces view diverse and/or similar colleagues as "being on the same team" or on different teams has strong implications for high productivity.

Many factors can cause diverse groups to be considered as part of a different team in healthcare workplaces. While the most simplistic answer is to assign all responses to implicit and/or explicit bias, the answer is far more complex. If the focus is only on the proximal, or most immediate causal variables, implicit and/or explicit bias possibly explain a large percentage of the failure to view all workers in healthcare workplaces as being on "one team." However, proximal causal analysis, in this case, references those variables within the present timeline that impacts workplace. However, underlying the proximal causes is another layer of variables which the healthcare community has labeled as *distal factors*.

Distal factors identify broader and more enduring variables that serve as the "soil" in which *proximal* causes grow. However, Liu et al. (2019) introduce the concept of the *Disparity Chain* as a tool for tracing the events that affect present-day outcomes over a larger historic period. The Disparity Chain seeks to map out the chain of causation into the known history and along interdisciplinary, cross-disciplinary, and transdisciplinary pathways within that historical milieu. This conceptual framework can be used to answer the question, "Why do some individuals and groups in healthcare and other workplaces not see culturally diverse workers as part of the overall team"? The answer is unique. Specifically, it supports the hypothesis that anthropological and historical illiteracy support various Isms that prevent all humans from being seen as a part of the same team both in workplaces and in general.

For example, anthropological illiteracy allows some workers to exclude their diverse colleagues from the overall "work team" because they are unaware of the specific anthropological findings that reveal the phase-by-phase process in which all humankind came from the same ancestors and spread across Earth's current landmasses. Knowing about the degree of resilience involved in this multimillion-year process creates a pride that would make any employee proud to be the "distant cousins" and "Teammates" of their workplace colleagues. Historical illiteracy prevents current-day healthcare and other workplace participants from feeling proud of the unique contributions of all anthropological "cousins" to the collective growth and development of humanity. For example, **TABLE 6.3** provides a brief overview of the exciting shared anthropological history of all humankind.

Understanding such simple anthropological information about the common origins of humankind has the power to transform diverse workplaces. Högberg and Gärdenfors (2015) discuss the relationship between what we know or think we know and the progression of humankind. These authors state "…human cooperation is distinctly extensive as a result of cumulative culture. Such cooperation may be uniquely reliant on an important mechanism – the human ability to teach our children—that is less frequently observed in other species" (page 113). This statement means that

TABLE 6.3 Why We're All Cousins: Key Points in the History of Humankind

Type of Development	Time Period	Factors Associated with the Change
1. The Emergence of Hominids.	2.5–4 million years ago in Eastern and Southern Africa	Climate and topological changes, etc.
2. The Emergence of homo habilis.	2.3 million years ago.	Increased brain capacity supported tool making, etc.
3. The hominid species Homo Erectus evolves and migrates out of Africa and into Eurasia.	1 million years ago.	Increased brain capacity allowed humankind to use fire and to engage in branching and speciation.
4. Homo Sapiens evolve.	200,000–300,000 years ago in Eastern and Northern Africa	Evolution to specific species.
5. Homo Sapiens become the only remaining hominids with 20,000 genes from one female, mtDNA, or mitochondrial Eve who lived in Africa around 200,000 years ago. mtDNA confirms that all Homo Sapiens have a common female ancestor.	150,000–200,000 years ago.	Humankind's struggle for resources, climate change, volcanic eruptions, etc.
6. Homo Sapiens migrate from Africa to Asia and Europe after a cognitive revolution.	Approximately 60,000–100,000 years ago	Making clothing from animal skins, making bows and arrows to hunt, constructing living quarters, etc.
7. Migration occurs to Australia, Europe.	35,000–45,000 years ago.	Humans' drive to survive.

8. Migration from Asia to Northern American continent by way of what is now Alaska.	13,000–14,000 years ago.	Ice Age created a land bridge.
9. The development of creative language.	70,000 years ago.	Cognitive growth.
10. The Agricultural Revolution.	12,000 years ago.	The shift from hunting and gathering to farming.
11. The development of Homo Sapien writings.	6,000 years ago in Mesopotamia.	Cognitive growth with use of tools.
12. The Scientific Revolution.	500 years ago.	Human curiosity.
13. The Industrial Revolution.	200–250 years ago.	Human curiosity and creativity, profit motive, etc.
14. The Information Revolution.	Late 1960s–Current.	Cognitive growth.
15. The Biotechnological Revolution.	1970s–Current.	Cognitive growth
16. The unity of Humankind Revolution.	Current.	Cognitive growth; alterations in ontology.

Data from Harari (2015), Sapiens: A Brief History of Humankind, New York: Harper; Rutherford, A. (2017). A Brief History of Everyone Who Ever Lived: The Human Story Retold Through Our Genes; and other sources; Poznik GD, Henn BM, Yee MC, Sliwerska E, Euskirchen GM, Lin AA, Snyder M, Quintana-Murci L, Kidd JM, Underhill PA, Bustamante CD (August 2013). "Sequencing Y chromosomes resolves discrepancy in time to common ancestor of males versus females." *Science, 341*(6145): 562–65. Cann, Rebecca L., et al. "Mitochondrial DNA and human evolution." Nature. January 1987. http://www.nature.com/nature/ancestor/pdf/325031.pdf. De Lorenzo, V. (2018). How biotechnology is evolving in the Fourth Industrial Revolution. Biotechnology. World Economic Forum. https://www.weforum.org/agenda/2018/05/biotechnology-evolve-fourth-industrial-revolution/

because we do not "teach our children" the common anthropological origins and interrelated pathways implicit to the development of humankind, these children, as adults, enter into their respective workplaces with no anthropological foundation. Yet, such a foundation is essential to respecting culturally diverse groups.

However, anthropological illiteracy also combines with historical illiteracy to prevent the maximization of outcomes in diverse workplaces via Isms. Historical illiteracy generates disrespect for culturally diverse populations in the workplace in the same way that low family socioeconomic status does. For example, Due et al. (2009), using a global sample of youth ages 11, 13, and 15 from nearly 6,000 schools in 35 countries, found that youth and adolescents who were believed to be from families of low socioeconomic status were at significantly higher risk of being bullied than their counterparts who were believed to be from a more affluent familial group. Historical illiteracy creates a parallel situation. That is, when illiteracy exists today regarding the historical socioeconomic status of various racial/ethnic, religious, and/or other culturally diverse groups in the workplace, cultural bullying presents itself as an internal and/or external bias against subgroups of workers. However, those who are historically literate understand that every single culturally diverse group has wealthy ancestors somewhere within their genealogical line. This historical fact is confirmed in **BOX 6.7**.

BOX 6.7   Sample of the Socioeconomic Status of Various Subgroups at Different Points in History

- Primary care physicians of Asian-Indian ethnicity encountered "bullying" and other forms of explicit and implicit bias in Great Britain as documented by Esmail (2007). Esmail documents that Asian-Indian physicians experienced wage/salary differentials, lack of access to patients other than those who lived in high-poverty areas and other disparities in labor market experience. While multiple variables exist, historical illiteracy is also at work.
- Medically, few healthcare workers are aware of Dr. Frederick Akbar Mohamed who is credited with the use of cohort studies today. Dr. Mohamed was a pioneer in introducing "collective investigation records" into medicine.
- Likewise, healthcare workers are historically illiterate regarding the high socioeconomic status achieved by Asian Indians over mankind's history, which includes events such as the Harappon cultures, which existed in 2500 BC; the Mauryan Empire (AD33 to 455); and others.
- Similarly, Ly et al. (2016), in an analysis of data for 43,213 physicians in workplaces in the United States, found that from 2010–2013, male physicians of African descent in the United States earned $64,812 less, on average, than male physicians of European descent. Bach et al. (2004) discovered that healthcare workers including physicians who serve African-American patients serve very few European-American patients. Norris (2013) interviewed an African-American physician, Dr. Gregory McGriff of North Carolina, who discussed the explicit distrust that he had encountered in the workplace with Caucasian patients.
- One may argue that this mistrust is generated, in part, by historical illiteracy regarding the "richness" of African culture. Historical illiteracy regarding African King Mansa Musa (Sullivan, 2016), who ruled from 1312 to 1337, was a key figure in the establishment of the University of Timbuktu. Mansa Musa had a net worth equivalent to $400 billion when measured in current dollars. Knowledge of him

alone would ameliorate beliefs regarding the low cultural capital among the ancestors of people of African descent who work in today's healthcare workplaces.

- Nunez-Smith (2009) analyzed the workplace experiences of 529 Asian Americans, Hispanic/Latino Americans, African Americans, and White Americans who indicated that workplace discrimination caused them to end their relationship with one or more healthcare institutions. Again, historical illiteracy regarding the great accomplishments of these culturally diverse populations may be a context for fewer assumptions of present day inferiority that emerge in contemporary workplaces. However, few workers in the healthcare environment are literate regarding Korean Kingdoms such as Samhan and/or the Chinese dynasties (Park, 2013; Gernet, 1996).

There are many other examples that confirm that diversity issues in healthcare workplaces today are related to anthropological and historical illiteracy among workers who endorse various Isms. While EEOC and/or cultural competency training can educate employees in healthcare environments regarding current workplace protection laws and/or introduce employees to the more contemporary folkways of diverse groups, the foundation of these Isms remains solid. Thus, such training alone will not address the untouched, very lengthy disparity chain that interacts to support problematic issues and conflict in culturally diverse workplaces today. HR Departments that use training as a tool may wish to shift the core elements that are used for cultural diversity and cultural competence training so that more foundational anthropological and/or historical illiteracy is also addressed.

The examples that are provided, although limited, do shift the focus from EEOC compliance and diversity training to promoting beliefs, attitudes, and behaviors in healthcare environments that promote humankind. Since all diverse groups of workers are human, such interventions will ultimately support a one-team workplace and the benefits that accrue from such an environment.

Positive Behavior Support or PBS (Sugai et al. 1997) is currently being used in special education. Sugai et al. define PBS as "…a general term that refers to the application of positive behavioral interventions and systems to achieve socially important behavior change" (page 6). The field of Behavioral Science asserts that "…much human behavior is learned, comes under the control of environmental factors, and can be changed" (Sugai et al. page 8). Applying this concept to healthcare workplaces, "…control of the behaviors" within the healthcare workplace can be changed via edutainment. Rather than the HR Department providing one workplace training session, an entire online "course" can be developed as a "soap" that literally uses edutainment to educate workers on the benefits of positive behavior within the workplace. The video, accompanied by a Toolkit of transmedia materials, can be used to inform and train people in the healthcare workplace on how the healthcare organization anticipates that workers and patients should be treated. The term "cultural diversity" would never be mentioned because such guidelines are not about diversity issues. The effort to reduce the presence of Isms in healthcare workplaces must focus on how human beings should treat other human beings. While there are many ethic-based ideals regarding how to treat other human beings, the most effective and rewarding criteria are for humans to be civil rather than uncivil. A workplace characterized by civilities will translate into the highest and greatest good for the whole of mankind.

Again, empirical evidence supports such an approach. Assche et al. (2018), in a study of 1,760 ethnically diverse individuals in Germany, found that "positive neighborhood norms" generated behaviors that offset negative behavior associated with past diversity issues. In order to triangulate these findings, a second study was completed with 993 Dutch adults. Again, positive neighborhood norms minimized the risks associated with diversity issues in the neighborhood. Nevertheless, the question can be asked. "But what suggests that persons with implicit and/or explicit bias against culturally diverse groups will cooperate with positive workplace norms"? Husnu and Paolini (2018) conducted a study that allowed conflicting ethnic groups in Turkey to engage in a visualization exercise based on very negative conflict between the groups and/or positive behavioral interactions. Most individuals from both groups chose visualizations based on positive interactions. This suggests that even in highly charged diverse work environments, all groups prefer positive intergroup interactions to negative ones.

▶ Reducing Isms in Healthcare Workplaces: Strategy #3 – Defining Augmented Roles for Human Resources Managers, Healthcare Administrators, Managers, and Employees

Human Resources Departments can be authorized by senior managers to adopt the use of transmedia, edutainment materials that promote positive interactions among all healthcare workers and the patients whom they serve. These materials can promote positive interactions such that every single behavior, action, or expression that is undertaken will increase human satisfaction. Positive interaction begins with an employee's attitudes, beliefs, and opinions regarding the nature of reality and finds expression in how that employee meets, greets, and generally interfaces with other employees and with the healthcare workplace's patients. To begin this process, workers will need to search within using therapeutic exercises such as those below:

- Describe your worst workplace experience.
- What made this experience so very unpleasant?
- Describe your best workplace experience.
- What made this experience so pleasant?

These searches also require other small group interchanges that allow each worker to better understand themselves. **BOX 6.8** provides an example of an instrument that can support self-understanding.

Second, a gradual movement to increase positive behavior in every area of life is slowly gaining momentum. Rather than focusing interventions on the existence of Isms, HR Departments, healthcare administrators, and managers may wish to start an internal campaign with different elements that focus on civility, community, and full workplace citizenship for all employees. The elements that are important to the success of a workplace can be included as part of a civility campaign.

Inadequate knowledge of the employer and the services and products that a healthcare workplace provides can create negative responses that cause negative

---

BOX 6.8 Understanding Your Own Attitudes, Opinions, and Beliefs

- Do you believe that a strong self-concept supports positive workplace experiences? Provide examples of how a strong self-concept can cause you to behave more positively in the workplace.
- Do you believe that an optimistic outlook regarding life will support positive workplace experiences? Provide examples of how an optimistic outlook can affect how you interface with your colleagues and with patients.
- Do you believe that feeling in control of your life can generate positive interactions with other workers and with patients? Provide an example of how not feeling in control of yourself can affect your workplace behavior.
- Do you have faith in the basic goodness of humanity? Provide examples of how faith in the basic goodness of humanity can affect your workplace interactions.
- In your lifetime, do you feel that you have had disproportionately positive life experiences? Provide examples of some of the positive life experiences that you would like to duplicate.
- In general, do you have a hopeful outlook? Provide examples of how a hopeful outlook can affect your interactions with colleagues and patients.
- Do you feel occupational and personal pride? Provide examples of how your personal pride has affected your interactions with colleagues and/or patients.
- Do you still feel excitement about your job? Provide examples of how excitement about your job can affect your interactions with your colleagues and with patients.
- Would you list any other attitudes, opinions, and beliefs that you feel affect whether you positively interact with your colleagues and patients?

---

behavior. Healthcare employers must include support for each employee's knowledge-base regarding positive workforce and patient relationships. Each worker must know not only his or her position but requirements for aspects of other workplace positions as well. Each worker must also understand how the healthcare industry is organized, how the healthcare environment functions best, and the products and services that are delivered in each healthcare workplace for maximum productivity. This will allow workers to be able to repeatedly study the workplace to provide the best care possible.

However, workers will also need training to develop positive worker traits and positive workplace interactions. Many characteristics can generate positive workplace interactions. Some of these include attitudes of enthusiasm, optimism, and professionalism while maintaining high performance. A commitment to the patient and the willingness to work hard to achieve the organization's goals are also critical behaviors. Through day-to-day interactions, positivity in the workplace means committing to credibility, friendliness, honesty, nonaggressiveness, politeness, reliability, responsibility, flexibility, resilience, sensitivity, and openness.

Positivity in the workplace is reinforced by displaying pleasant, interpersonal, and polite communication skills including the ability to engage in active listening. Asking effective questions is also important. Demonstrating that a person understands a colleague's needs perpetuates positivity in the workplace. Also, being able to communicate politely and clearly without resorting to negative behaviors such as sarcasm, blame, etc., are key. As is true for a sports team, conflict is reduced and respect is generated when each worker prepares for his or her job by preparing for each task. Positive workplace interactions require that each worker be less reactive and more proactive. Workers should not compete to be harder working than their peers. Rather, each employee should do the very best they can do. If employees demonstrate this type of behavior, we anticipate that more positive human interactions will extend beyond the workplace. Additionally, the transmedia edutainment workplace training activities can demonstrate strategies to support relationship-building. In so doing, healthcare administrators, HR managers, and other managers can expand findings to generate changes in human interactions in the workplace that reduce Isms and, as a result, increase productivity.

Rahimi et al. (2017) summarize some of the human relations skills that have been used in tourism and hospitality. The same strategies can be used by workers in healthcare places and other workplaces as well as with patients. Excellent "customer service skills" can become the standard for human encounters. It is important, however, that healthcare workers do not mistake all criticisms as an Ism. To increase productivity, workers must be open to criticism. It is necessary to have supervision and monitoring in the workplace. However, supervisors can use a gentle, civil approach in providing criticism of the work performed.

Similarly, managers can be trained to manage issues, not people. Getting into a verbal or nonverbal confrontation with other people is never acceptable nor conducive to higher productivity. Employees can be trained to interact positively with others and to eliminate routinely negative interactions. The training will teach employees to interact positively with their colleagues, which will promote workplace harmony. Employees must also be active, attentive participants in any conversation and be responsive to other people without dominating the conversation. Such behavior in healthcare workplaces discourages behaviors associated with Isms or other negative causes.

Verbal communication is used every day between healthcare coworkers to achieve their common work goals. Verbal communication is used to describe tasks, ask and answer questions, summarize procedures and findings, and discuss and brainstorm health-related matters and ideas. However, workers may need training on how to communicate to avoid any misunderstandings. Trager (1958) coined the term "paralanguage" to describe certain characteristics of verbal communication including the tone, volume, pauses, inflection, and other characteristics of human speech that can convey messages without words. These characteristics can mean different things across cultures. For example, speaking in a low tone to a patient could be interpreted as a sign of respect in the United States or humility in another country (Crezee et al. 2016). Researchers Stivers et al. (2009) studied "turn-taking" among different cultures and found that Danish people had the slowest response times in conversation and that Japanese participants had the fastest response times. In an article that includes paralanguage, Pennycock (1985) suggests that these types of communication differences be addressed in cultural competency training.

In diverse healthcare and other workplaces, one culprit that can serve as a source of conflict is **nonverbal communication**. In the book, *Nonverbal Communications in Human Interactions*, Knapp, Hall, and Horgan (2013) provide a detailed description of how humans interpret various forms of nonverbal communication. No eye contact can be considered as an incivility among healthcare workers in the United States. Shiota et al. (2017), for example, examine the different types of positive emotions and how these can be "constructed." Mehrabian (2007) describes how positive facial expressions and other nonverbal signs convey messages to others. He suggests that the most often used nonverbal tools include: 1) the degree of the contact; 2) the physical distance between two people; 3) the type of facial expressions; 4) positions of people's feet and legs; and 5) other cues. According to Mehrabian, however, considered together, these and other nonverbal signals are often used to communicate messages regarding the degree of positivity and/or negativity that the individual is feeling. Such behaviors also signify social status that the individual has assigned to the person or persons to whom such nonverbal cues are directed. Finally, Mehrabian indicates that these behaviors communicate the overall responsiveness of one individual to another. **BOX 6.9** provides some tips on essential nonverbal behaviors.

Again, educating workers in culturally diverse workplaces to findings such as these also reduces diversity-related conflict by training healthcare workers to be more "human" to each other and to the patients they serve.

BOX 6.9 Nonverbal Communications

- Words transmit a small percentage of information even when exchanged face-to-face (Thompson, 2011).
- Voice characteristics contribute to face-to-face messages, but most of the messages are received based on body language, appearances, and related factors (Thompson, 2011).
- If one uses back-and-forth motions when interfacing with a person, it indicates insecurity (Navarro, 2011). However, side-to-side motions while interacting with a person indicates a positive outlook.
- When a person leans forward toward the person, the body language suggests a positive response (Study-body-language.com).
- If a person leans away from the other person, it indicates boredom or self-protection (McKay, Davis & Fanning, 2018).
- A person can tell if the other person is truly interested in him or her because the person's pupils will enlarge (Navarro, 2018).
- Intense eye contact for more than 1 or 2 seconds can be regarded as an impolite gesture (Navarro, 2018).
- A gaze to the right indicates that the person is responding to the logic and facts of the information shared by the individual (simplybodylanguage.com).
- A gaze to the left indicates more intense concentration based on emotional or memory responses (simplybodylanguage.com).
- Tightness of the cheek, jaw line, or neck suggests tension and anger (Navarro, 2018).
- Broad and vigorous arm movements imply that the person is emphatic about the point being communicated (Navarro, 2018).
- Self-touching by the individual suggests self-comforting (Navarro, 2018). However, tense crossing of the arms can be a sign of insecurity or as a form of protection.
- Intertwined or steepled hands suggest assurance and confidence (Navarro, 2018).
- If the person's legs are uncrossed and in an open position, it symbolizes cooperation, confidence, and comfort (Navarro, 2018).
- Crossed legs toward a person indicates acceptance (Smith, 2015).
- People should pay attention to proximity and personal space when engaging with others so as not to make the other person feel uncomfortable or threatened (Navarro, 2018).
- First personal contact should be limited to a handshake (Navarro, 2018).

(continues)

BOX 6.9 Nonverbal Communications   *(continued)*

- Open and relaxed hands suggest that the person is responding positively. This is particularly true if palms are facing up, which indicate peace and cooperation. This gesture serves also to show the absence of weapons (studybodylanguage.com).
- However, body language must also be culturally interpreted. For example, Tidwell (2016) indicates that in many cultures, avoiding eye contact can be a sign of respect. In Middle Eastern countries and Thailand, it is considered an insult to show the bottom of one's shoe or foot (the dirtiest and lowest part of your body). In Northern European countries, slumping or poor posture can be considered rude behavior.

Constructed by the Authors from information sources cited.

▶ Reducing Isms in Healthcare Workplaces: Strategy #4 – The Issue of Clothing and Hairstyles

Campbell (2018) reports on a company called Catastrophe Management Solutions that, in 2013, offered a position to an African-American female from Alabama that was contingent on her "cutting her dreadlocks." She sued the company and the claim was dismissed. The issue made its way to the Supreme Court, which chose not to rule on the case. However, as stated in Chapter 1, in early July, 2019, California became the first state to ban hairstyle discrimination through the "Crown Act" (SB 188). The "Crown Act" has also passed the Senate in New York State and has been introduced to New Jersey lawmakers. Dove, with partners, National Urban League, Color Of Change, and Western Center on Law, and Poverty, founded the Creating a Respectful and Open World for Natural Hair (CROWN Coalition).

In a recent Dove survey, their researchers found that only 20% of African Americans were unlikely to alter their natural hair in order to adhere to workplace expectations (Dove, 2019). Additionally, the survey found that half of the African-American female respondents had either been asked to return home due to their hairstyle or knew of someone who had received the same request from their employer (ibid).

Scafidi (2017) describes evidence that people working in culturally diverse workplaces are aggressively seeking legal remedies to workplaces that define work attire standards. However, the mandatory use of uniforms remains legal as long as the uniforms are not differentiated by sex. This raises the question of whether the manner of dress affects high productivity in healthcare and other workplaces or if prescribed dress and hairstyles associated with adverse beliefs, attitudes, and behaviors can reflect the assumption of superiority or inferiority?

Dress and overall workplace appearance affect productivity. In a study of 201 male and female dentists and lawyers, Furnham (2013) found that the clients of lawyers and dentists prefer more formal dress. Landry et al. (2013) analyzed patients' preferences regarding how their physicians "should" dress. Approximately 84% of patients in hospital clinics and 51.9% of patients in hospitals preferred their physician to wear white coats with shirts below their elbows.

In response to current issues regarding workplace attire in a culturally diverse world, Sulanke et al. (2015) conducted a study that could be used to reconcile patients' preferences with potential dress code changes. With this goal in mind, an Image of Nursing Subcommittee was established. A comprehensive literature review was conducted. Additionally, key nursing organizations were contacted. Survey data were also collected from nurses and current or past patients. The findings were most informative. First, a consensus supported the need for attire to make nurses easily identifiable. Second, patients associated greater professionalism with better care. Yet, nurses wanted to ensure that their clothing was supportive of their duties. Other findings were also revealed.

The preferences of the public regarding clothing and overall dress of workers is linked with organizational profitability and, in some instances, wages and salaries. Kiisel (2013) summarized other research, which reveals that dress and physical appearance generate greater revenue streams to the individuals and to their employers. Accordingly, one may argue that dress and hairstyle codes in healthcare workplaces can be legitimately prescribed and do not necessarily reflect the existence of Isms in healthcare workplaces.

William Shakespeare wrote, "All the world's a stage, and all the men and women merely players." Such a statement is particularly applicable to the workplace. Workplaces, whether for profit and/or not-for-profit, must maximize their productivity to provide goods and/or services. Productivity cannot be maximized without delivering to consumers the type of "goods" and services desired, in the place desired, at the price desired, and with the characteristics desired. The owners or administrators of organizations are charged with the duty of guaranteeing the survival of the organization. With that goal in mind, they can conduct research and provide the "marketing mix" that will support the survival of the organization. This process includes a "Script" and a "Stage." Each work environment then "Casts" for the various roles, defines the "Wardrobes" that will best resonate with their "audience," and "directs" the delivery of lines as well as other aspects of the "production." Thus, the "actors" (workers) do not and should not have the power to define the "character." However, they do have the power to audition for parts in a different play and on a different stage. Stated more directly, high productivity in a diverse workplace requires cooperation and accommodation for all. Perhaps the issue of dress and overall physical attire should be considered by diverse workers before accepting employment in an industry with incompatible "wardrobe" requirements. However, as our previous discussion on "lookism" suggests, employees should not be forced to change their natural appearance to be employed and it seems that government agencies are starting to take steps to protect a natural appearance.

▶ Summary

The theme of this book is Isms in healthcare workplaces. This chapter provides some alternative approaches to higher productivity in diverse workplaces. It began by introducing the idea that present-day human interactions in diverse workplaces that are based on competition and conflict are incompatible with productivity. It then introduced disparity chain analysis to argue that anthropological and historical illiteracy are partly responsible for some diverse groups being considered "inferior" to other groups.

The argument was then made that the remediation of competition and competitiveness in culturally diverse workplaces requires interventions that generate improved human interactions in the workplace. Subsequently, positive behaviors and, as a result, maximum productivity in healthcare and other workplaces were determined. Competition and conflict in culturally diverse workplaces can be eliminated if each trained employee embodies the following traits: a strong self-concept; an optimistic outlook on life; an internal locus of control; faith in the basic goodness of humanity; mostly positive life experiences; a hopeful outlook; occupational and personal pride; excitement about the job; patience, sensitivity, and understanding; a calm demeanor; friendliness; openness; politeness; honesty; and credibility.

Healthcare workplaces are already positioned to heal. This healing can be directed to the workplace itself by ensuring that individual workers use a framework that understands that *oneness* is the objective of the world today. The noted genius, Stephen Hawking, hypothesized that the Earth will be "burned away in one century." Therefore, residents must work collectively as a whole to create a new future. Applying behavioral change strategies to ensure that employees self-analyze and confront their own attitudes and behaviors to support a workplace characterized by cooperation and accommodation is key. A workplace that is inclusionary and in which everyone is working toward the same goal does, indeed, have a higher probability of higher productivity.

Wrap-Up

Review Questions

1. Support or oppose the following statement, "If a healthcare workplace remains in 100% compliance with EEOC regulations, the HR Department shall have reduced the adverse impact of Isms in that workplace."
2. Explain whether the statement that follows is true or false and why: "Cultural competency training is the most powerful tool available for the HR Department to use in reducing the adverse impact of Isms upon output maximization in healthcare workplaces."
3. The adoption of behaviors that exclude incivilities in healthcare workplaces will support reduced adverse beliefs, attitudes, and behaviors. Explain this statement.

Key Terms and Concepts

Cortisol

DHEA

Diversity Dimensions

EEOC

External Directives

Investigational Directives

Nonverbal Communications

Unconstrained Inclusion

References

Allen, R. S., Dawson, G. D., Wheatley, K., & White, C. S. (2008). Perceived diversity and organizational performance. *Employee Relations, 30*(1), 20–33. doi:10.1108/01425450810835392

Arnold, P. (2011). The role of diversity management in the global talent retention race. *Profiles in Diversity Journal,* http://www.diversityjournal.com/4530-the-role-of-diversity-management -in-the-global-talent-retention-race/. May 27, 2011.

Assche, J., Asbrock, F., Roets, A., & Kauff, M. (2018). Positive neighborhood norms buffer ethnic diversity effects on neighborhood dissatisfaction, perceived neighborhood disadvantage, and moving intentions. *Personality & Social Psychology Bulletin, 44*(5), 700–716. doi: 10.01461672177447667

Bach, P. B., Pham, H. H., Schrag, D., Tate, R. C., & Hargraves, J. L. Primary care physicians who treat blacks and whites. *New England Journal of Medicine, 351*(6), 575–584. doi:10.1056 /NEJMsa040609

Banks, K. H. (2016). How managers can promote healthy discussions about race. *Harvard Business Review*, January 7, 2016. https://hbr.org/2016/01/how-managers-can-promote-healthy -discussions-about-race

Campbell, A. F. (2018). A black woman lost a job offer because she wouldn't cut her dreadlocks, now she wants to go to the Supreme Court. *Vox*, https://www.vox.com/2018/4/18/17242788 /chastity-jones-dreadlock-job-discrimination.

Cann, R. L., Stoneking, M., & Wilson, A. C. (1987). Mitochondrial DNA and human evolution. *Nature*, 325, 31–36.

Carrè, J. M., Geniole, S. N., Ortiz, T. L., Bird, B. M., Videto, A., & Bonin, P. L. (2017). Exogenous testosterone rapidly increases aggressive behavior in dominant and impulsive men. *Biological Psychiatry, 82*(4), 249–256. doi:10.1016/j.biopsych.2016.06.009

Catalyst. Engaging in conversations about gender, race, and ethnicity in the workplace. (2016) Catalyst's Women of Color Research Agenda: New Approaches, New Solutions. New York: Catalyst. http://www.catalyst.org/system/files/engaging_in_conversations_about_gender_race _and_ethnicity_in_the_workplace.pdf

Chua, A., & Rubenfeld, J. (2014). The triple package how three unlikely traits explain the rise and fall of cultural groups in America. Penguin Press HC. P. 53. ISBN 978-159425460.

Crezee, I. H. M., Gailani, N., & Gailani, A. N. (2016). Introduction to healthcare for Arabic-speaking interpreters and translators. Page 25 Johns Benjamins Publishing Company: Amsterdam/ Philadelphia.

De Lorenzo, V. (2018). How biotechnology is evolving in the Fourth Industrial Revolution. Biotechnology. *World Economic Forum*, https://www.weforum.org/agenda/2018/05 /biotechnology-evolve-fourth-industrial-revolution/

Desai, S. D., Chugh, D., & Brief, A. P. (2014). The implications of marriage structure for men's workplace attitudes, beliefs, and behaviors toward women. *Administrative Science Quarterly, 59*(2), 330–365. doi:10.1177/0001839214528704

Deutsch, D. (2005). The psychology of music. Waltham, MA: Academic Press.

Dobbin, F., Schrage, D., & Kalev, A. (2015). Rage against the iron cage—*The varied effects of bureaucratic personnel reforms on diversity. American Sociological Review, 80*(5), 1014–1044. September 1, 2015. doi:10.1177/0003122415596416

Dove. The Crown Coalition. (2019) Cision PR Newswire May 1, 2019. New Dove study confirms workplace bias against hairstyles impacts Black women's ability to celebrate their natural beauty: Dove co-founds CROWN Coalition to push for legislation to end hair discrimination at work and in schools. https://www.prnewswire.com/news-releases/new-dove-study-confirms -workplace-bias-against-hairstyles-impacts-black-womens-ability-to-celebrate-their-natural -beauty-300842006.html

Due, P., Merlo, J., Harel-Fisch, Y., Damsgaard, M. T., Holstein, B. E., Hetland, J., … Lynch, J. (2009). Socioeconomic inequality in exposure to bullying during adolescence: A comparative, cross sectional multilevel study in 35 countries. *American Journal of Public Health, 99*(5), 907–914. doi:10.2105/AJPH.2008.139303

Eagly, A. H. (2016). When passionate advocates meet research on diversity, does the honest broker stand a chance? *Journal of Social Issues, 72*(1). doi:10.1111/josi.12163

Edwards, L. (2010). Estimate of flowering plant species to be cut by 600,000. https://phys.org/news/2010-09-species.html Retrieved Monday, June 4, 2018.

EEOC (2020). Charge Statistics (Charges Filed with EEOC) FY 1997 Through FY 2019. https://www.eeoc.gov/eeoc/statistics/enforcement/charges.cfm

EEOC Press Releases at https://www.eeoc.gov/eeoc/newsroom/release/

Esmail, A. (2007). Asian doctors in the NHS: Service and betrayal. *British Journal of General Practice, 57*(543), 827–834. PMC2151817

Furnham, A., Chan, P. S., & Wilson, E. (2014). What to wear: The influence of attire on the perceived professionalism of dentists and lawyers. *Journal of Applied Social Psychology, 43*(9), 1838–1859, doi:10.111.asp.12136

Gernet, J. (1996). A history of Chinese civilization. Cambridge University Press, p. 420.

Goldbach, J. (2017). Diversity toolkit: A guide to discussing identity, power and privilege. USC Suzanne Dworak-Peck School of Social Work. https://msw.usc.edu/mswusc-blog/diversity-workshop-guide-to-discussing-identity-power-and-privilege/

Harari, Y. (2015). Sapien: A brief history of humankind. New York: Harper.

Hardcastle, S. J., & Hagger, M. S. (2015). Psychographic profiling for effective health behavior change interventions. *Frontiers in Psychology, 6*:1988. Published online 2016 Jan 6. doi:10.3389/fpsyg.2015.01988

Herring, C. (2009). Does diversity pay? Race, gender, and the business case for diversity. *American Sociological Review, 74*(2), 208–224, doi:10.1177/000312240907400203

Högberg, A., & Gärdenfors, P. (2015). Children, teaching and the evolution of humankind. *Childhood in the Past, 8*(2), 113–121. doi:10/1179/1758571615Z,000000000033

Hoobler, J. M., Masterson, C. R., Nkomo, S. M., & Michel, E. J. (2016). The business case for women leaders: Meta-analysis, research critique, and path forward. *Journal of Management, 44*(6), 2473–2499. doi:10.1177/0149206316628643

Husnu, S., & Paolini, S. (2018). Positive imagined contact is actively chosen: Exploring determinants and consequences of volitional intergroup imagers in a conflict-ridden setting. *Group Processes and Interagency Relations*, 1–19. doi:10.1177/1368430217747405

Jernigan, V. B. B., Hearod, J. B., Tran, K., Norris, K. C., & Buchwald, D. (2016). An examination of cultural competence training in US medical education guided by the tool for assessing cultural competence training. *Journal of Health Disparities Research Practice, 9*(3), 150–167.

Kedem, M. (2016). Don't shy away from discussing difficult topics of race and equity at work. World Changing Ideas. Fast Company. https://www.fastcompany.com/3062571/your-work-should-make-it-easy-to-discuss-difficult-topics-of-race-and-equity-at-the-office

Kiisel, T. (2013). You are judged by your appearance. *Forbes*, https://www.forbes.com/sites/tykiisel/2013/03/20/you-are-judged-by-your-appearance/#d66f5326d50c

Knapp, M. L., Hall, J. A., & Horgan, T. G. (2014). Nonverbal communication in human interaction. Wadsworth: Boston, MA.

Landry, M., Dornelles, A. C., Hayek, G., & Deichmann, R. E. (2013). Patient preferences for doctor attire: The white coat's place in the medical profession. *The Oschsner Journal, 13*(3), 334–342.

Lepak, D. P., & Snell, S. A. (1999). The human resource architecture: Toward a theory of human capital allocation and development, *The Academy of Management Review, 24*(1), 31–48. doi:10.2307/259035

Liu, D., Burston, B., Collier-Stewart, S., & Mulligan, H. H. (2018). The challenges of health disparities: Implications and actions for health care professionals. Jones & Bartlett Learning: Burlington: MA.

Ly, D. P., Seabury, S. A., & Jena, A. B. (2016). Differences in incomes of physicians in the United States by race and sex: Observational study. *British Medical Journal*, 353, i2923. doi:10.1136/bmj.12923

MacDonald, R. A. R. (2013). Music, health, and well-being: A review. *International Journal of Quality Studies on Health and Well-being*, 8, 20635. 10.3402/qhw.v8i0.20635. https://www.ncbi.nlm.nih.gov/pmc/articles/PMC3740599/

Martin, G. C. The effects of cultural diversity in the workplace. (2014). *Journal of Diversity Management, 9*(2). doi:10.19020/jdm.v9j2.8974

McHale, T. S., Chee, W., Chan, K. C., Zava, D. T., & Gray, P. B. (2018). Coalitional physical competition: Acute salivary steroid hormone responses among juvenile male soccer players in Hong Kong. *Human Nature, 29*(3), 245–267. doi:10.1007/s12110-018-9321-7

McKay, M., Davis, M., & Fanning, P. (2018). Messages: The communication skills book. 4th Ed. Oakland, CA: New Harbinger Publications, Inc.

Mehrabian, A. (2017) Nonverbal Communication. (first published 1972) New York: Routledge.

Navarro, J. (with Poynter, T.S.) (2011) (originally published 1953). Louder than words: take your career from average to exceptional with the hidden power of nonverbal intelligence. Harper Collins Publishers: New York.

Navarro, J. (2018). The dictionary of body language: A field guide to human behavior. New York: NY: William Morrow.

Norris, M. (2013). For a black doctor, building trust by slowing down. *National Public Radio*, https://www.npr.org.

Nunez-Smith, M., Pilgrim, N., Wynia, M., Desai, M. M., Bright, C., Krumholz, H. M., & Bradley, E. H. (2009). Health care workplace discrimination and physician turnover, *Journal of the National Medical Association, 101*(12), 1274–1282.

Park, S-H (2013). Changing definitions of sovereignty in nineteenth-century east Asia: Japan and Korea between China and the west. *Journal of East Asian Studies, 13*(2), 281–307. doi:10.1017/S1598240800003945

Pennycock, A. (1985) Actions speak louder than words: Paralanguage, communication and education. *TESOL Quarterly, 19*(2), 259–282. doi:10.2307/3586829

Poznik, G. D., Henn, B. M., Yee, M. C., Sliwerska, E., Euskirchen, G. M., Lin, A. A., Snyder, M., Quintana-Murci, L., Kidd, J. M., Underhill, P. A., & Bustamante, C. D. (August 2013). "Sequencing Y chromosomes resolves discrepancy in time to common ancestor of males versus females." *Science, 341*(6145): 562–65.

Prasad, S., Narayanan, J., Lim, V. K. G., Koh, G. C. H., Koh, D. S. Q., & Mehta, P. H. (2017). Preliminary evidence that acute stress moderates basal testosterone's association with retaliatory behavior. *Hormones and Behavior, 92*, 128–140. doi:10.1016/j.yhbeh.2016.10.020

Rahimi, R., Köseoglu, M. A., Ersoy, A. B., & Okumus, F. (2017). Customer relationship management research on tourism and hospitality: A state-of-the-art. *Tourism Review, 72*(2), 209–220. doi:10.1108/TR-01-2017.0011

Rentfrow, P. J. (2012). The role of music in everyday life: Current directions in the social psychology of music. *Social and Personality Psychology Compass, 6*(5). doi:10.1111/j.1751-9004.2012.00434.x

Richard, O. C. (2000). Racial diversity, business strategy; and firm performance: A resource-based view. *Academy of Management Journal, 43*(2), 164–177. doi:10.2307/1556374

Rutherford, A. (2017). A brief history of everyone who ever lived: The human story retold through our genes. The Experiment. LLC.

Scafidi, S. (2017). Think Tank: Is your company's dress code illegal? *WWD*, https://wwd.com/business-news/business-features/think-tank-susan-scafidi-dress-codes-10853345/

Schäfer, T. (2016). The goals and effects of music listening and their relationship to the strength of music preference. *PLoS One, 11*(3): e0151634. Published online 2016 Mar 17. doi:10.1371/journal.pone.0151634

Shiota, M. N., Campos, B., Oveis, C., Hertenstein, M. J., Simon-Thomas, E., & Keltner, D. (2017). Beyond happiness: Building a science of discrete positive emotions. *American Psychologist, 72*(7), 617–643. doi:10/1037/a0040456

Simply Body Language.com: Body language without the psycho-babble. Eye body language: Reading basic eye movements. https://www.simplybodylanguage.com/eye-body-language.html

Smith, A. (2017). Top 10 Employment Cases of 2017 Reviewed. Society for Human Resource Management—SHRM. Conference Today. https://www.shrm.org/hr-today/news/hr-news/conference-today/pages/2017/top-10-employment-cases-of-2017-reviewed.aspx, Jun 19, 2017.

Smith, S. (2015). What is your body language saying? Realsimple.com. https://www.realsimple.com/health/mind-mood/reading-body-language?

Soga, M., Gaston, K. J., & Yamaura, Y. (2017). Gardening is beneficial for health: A meta-analysis. *Preventative Medicine Reports, 5*:92–99.

Stanford Encyclopedia of Philosophy. Wednesday, May 30, 2018. Logic and Information, https://plato.stanford.edu.

Stivers, T., Enfield, N. J., Brown, P., Englert, C., Hayashi, M., Heinemann, T., ... Levinson, S. C. (2009). Universal and cultural variation in turn-taking in conversation. *PNAS, 106*(26), 10587–10592. doi:10.1073/pnas.0903616106

Study Body Language. http://www.study-body-language.com/

Sugai, G., Horner, R. H., Dunlap, G., Hieneman, M., Lewis, T. J., Nelson, C. M., ... Ruef, M. Applying positive behavior support and functional behavioral assessments in schools. *Journal of Positive Behavioral Interventions, 2*(3), 131–143. doi:10.1177/109830070000200302

Sulanke, J., & Shimp, K. (2015). What works: Implementing an evidence-based nursing dress code to enhance professional image. *American Nurse, 10*(10). https://www.americannursetoday.com/works-implementing-evidence-based-nursing-dress-code-enhance-professional-image/

Sullivan, K. (2016). Mansa Musa: The richest man in history. https://www.ancient-origins.net/history-famous-people/mansa-musa-richest-man-history-006847

Thompson, J. (2011). Is nonverbal communication a numbers game? *Psychology Today*, https://www.psychologytoday.com/us/blog/beyond-words/201109/is-nonverbal-communication-numbers-game

Thurow, L. (1978). Psychic income: Useful or useless? *American Economic Review, 68*(2), 142–45.

Tidwell, C. (2016). Non-verbal communication modes. https://www.andrews.edu/~tidwell/bsad560/NonVerbal.html

Trager, G. L. (1958). Paralanguage: A first approximation. *Studies in Linguistics, 12*, 1–12. Department of Anthropology and Linguistics, University of Buffalo.

United States Bureau of the Census. Median household income in the past 12 months (and 2014 inflation-adjusted dollars). American Community Survey. United States Census Bureau. 2014. Retrieved December 3, 2015.

United States Bureau of the Census. Median household income in the past 12 months (and 2015 inflation-adjusted dollars). American Community Survey. United States Census Bureau. 2015. Retrieved December 3, 2016.

United States Equal Employment Opportunity Commission. https://www.eeoc.gov

United States Equal Employment Opportunity Commission. Charge Statistics National FY 1997–2019). https://www.eeoc.gov/eeoc/statistics/enforcement/charges.cfm

Wagner, J. D., Flinn, M. V., & England, B. G. (2002). Hormonal response to competition among male coalitions. *Evolution and Human Behavior, 23*(6), 437–442. doi:10.1016/S1090-5138(02)00100-9

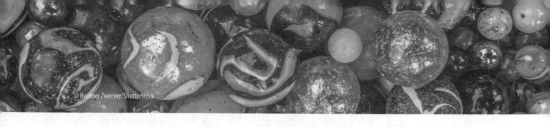

CHAPTER 7

Epilogue: Where Do We Go from Here?

"We are very, very small, but we are profoundly capable of very, very big things."

– Stephen Hawking (1942–2018), an English theoretical
physicist, cosmologist, and author

In 2016, there were 5,534 registered hospitals in the United States (American Hospital Association, 2018). In addition, as of 2015, there were 230,187 workplaces that were classified as physician/practices (Kane, 2015). The present day healthcare marketplace incudes nursing homes, assisted-living organizations, pharmacies, home-health agencies, hospices, public-health organizations, community-health centers, surgicenters, walk-in clinics, alternative medicine clinics, dialysis centers, rehabilitation centers, dental offices, and a host of other workplaces. More and more, these workplaces will recruit, hire, manage, assess, promote, and employ workers who are two or more standard deviations from the characteristics that have, in the past, represented the central tendency for the American labor market in general and for healthcare marketplaces in particular.

Johnson (February 14, 2018), for example, reported that while only 17.6% of physicians aged 65 and older are female, 60.6% of physicians under age 35, and 51.5% of physicians in the age group 35–44 are female. While the population in general may continue to believe that physicians are a male-dominated profession, in healthcare workplaces of the future, this is not the case. Similarly, data from the Kaiser Family Foundation (October 2018) reveal that while males only comprise 9% of all nurses, the absolute number of nurses who classify themselves as males exceeds 333,530 people. One study reported that 3.8% of the population classified themselves as gay, lesbian, transgender, or bisexual (Flores, 2018). By 2015, this percentage had increased to 4.5% (Fitzsimons, 2018). However, an estimated 7.3% of people whose birth years were from 1980–1998 describe themselves as LGBT (Allen, 2017). Braithwaite (March 10, 2016) reported that a study by the J. Walter Thompson Innovation Group discovered that only 48% of the 13 to 20 years old sampled described themselves as 100% heterosexual. Accordingly, existing central tendency-ism in workplaces throughout the United States relative to heterosexism is changing.

Hanes (June 13, 2015) discusses data that suggest that sexualism may actually increase as an issue in healthcare and other workplaces. This is because the number of Americans who are unmarried currently outnumber those who are married. Moreover, one study (Trustify, 2018), completed a small convenience survey of almost 200 people. Approximately 80% of males and 36% of females responded positively to a query regarding their participation in marital infidelity. Moreover, approximately 55% of the males surveyed had been sexually involved with five or more people. In many cases, the initiation of these sexualisms, independent of marital status, occur in the workplace.

Current data also suggest that IQism has the potential to become an even greater threat in healthcare and other workplaces. Cannabis use for medicinal and/or recreational use has been legalized in a number of states. Moreover, data from the Centers for Disease Control and Prevention's Youth Risk Behavior Surveillance System (YRBSS) survey reveal that in 2007, approximately 19.7% of high school students indicated current marijuana use. However, by 2017, this number had fluctuated to 19.8% from a high of 23.4% in 2013. Approximately 1/5 of high school students currently use marijuana and have done so for the past 10 years. Becker et al. (2018), using a before and after design, assessed changes in verbal learning and memory, and motivated decision making, planning, and working memory in frequent cannabis users over 2 years. The study revealed a number of impairments in key areas that are associated with IQ measurements. These and future youth now represent the pool from which future healthcare and nonhealthcare workers will be drawn. Thus, environmental, sociopolitical, and cultural changes are occurring within the context of the many other forces that have already supported decreases in the central tendency for IQ within the United States. Bratsberg and Rogeberg (2018) reference the fact that IQs in Norway, the United States, and other countries first increased during the 20th century and then began to decrease. Moreover, they argue that such trends were occurring within families and not between families. Dockrill (June 13, 2018) summarizes research from scholarly studies that reveal that overall IQ is decreasing. Such circumstances can increase the potential for IQism in healthcare and other workplaces.

Healthcare workplaces are now more diverse than ever. However, they are also in need of greater diversity. For example, while approximately 75% of Native Americans have health insurance, they are extremely underrepresented in American healthcare workplaces. Gray (2016) reports that as recently as 2015, only 20, or 0.1%, of the 8,000 medical school graduates embodied the level of understanding of one or more Native American culture that coincides with birth and nurturance by that culture. Stated differently, only 20 of these medical school graduates had a comprehensive understanding of the ways of life that may affect the health of one or more Native American tribes as a result of their history and tradition. Likewise, Ambrose et al. (2012) documented similar circumstances for Native Hawaiians and, particularly, for other Pacific Islanders. An article published by the Associated Press (October 8, 2016) suggests that as workplaces, Native-American hospitals themselves are characterized by numerous human variables that prevent high productivity.

Thus, when the issues covered in this text, i.e., IQism, sexualism, heterosexism, etc., are analyzed separately, it becomes clear that many forces are major threats to productivity in healthcare workplaces. However, these threats are enhanced because various "Isms" in American healthcare workplaces do not operate in isolation. Rather, as a result of intersectionalities, these and other "Isms" operate in many different ways. Accordingly, the impact on the productivity of healthcare workplaces can be extremely negative. Thus, while the purpose of this primer is to advance understanding of how the discussed Isms function, it is also important to explore these forces within the context of dialogue surrounding the question, "How can the future of humankind be advanced by moving past central tendencyism and advancing output maximization by reducing the operations of these and other Isms in healthcare workplaces"?

Ali et al. (2018) demonstrate that "…a higher level of human capital can affect productivity if it is efficiently utilized by the economic state" (page 2). In other words, the nature and effective operation of social systems and institutions interfere with the relationship between human capital and maximum economic output from available resources. The argument has been taken further in this Handbook that humankind in healthcare and other workplaces are allowing uncivil responses to human dispersion and useless efforts to enforce central tendencyism to locate human achievements far below their potential. While such an argument can be applied generally, the impact of such behaviors are magnified when they occur in healthcare workplaces and in education-delivering workplaces. Stated differently, when high productivity is undermined in the very "factories" that produce human capital—health and education—the entirety of the progress of humankind is stymied, delayed, and, in some cases, reversed. Accordingly, solutions are sorely needed.

We, the authors, cannot say where healthcare administrators and workers and other leaders of human capital institutions "ought-to-and-or-should-go." By concentrating on strengthening the country's healthcare systems and making them more efficient, productivity can be maximized. We also know that through the identification of and addressing of Central Tendencyism, the United States can look forward to a healthcare workforce that maximizes its output. We know that by decreasing negative behaviors in healthcare workplaces, the healthcare services provided to the people will improve. We have made some suggestions for each of the "Isms" analyzed in this primer. However, neither government agencies nor healthcare administrators and managers alone can generate the level of changes needed. Maximizing productivity in healthcare and other workplaces will start with each individual exploring his or her day-to-day actions and asking, "Did I apply civilities in every area of my gross and nuanced behavior"? By behaving positively, healthcare and other workplaces can be transformed and humankind can creatively search for the solutions change the future. Those changes start with each one of us.

References

Ali, M., Egbetokun, A., & Memon, M. H. (2018). Human capital, social capabilities and economic growth. *Economies*, https://www.mdpi.com/2227-7099/6/1/2/pdf

Allen, S. (January 14, 2017). Counted Out: Just how many LGBT Americans are there? *Daily Beast*, https://www.thedailybeast.com/just-how-many-lgbt-americans-are-there

Ambrose, A. J. H., Arakawa, R. Y., Greidanus, B. D., Macdonald, P. R., Racsa, C. P., Shibuya, K. T., … Yamada, S. (2012). Geographical maldistribution of Native Hawaiian and other Pacific Islander Physician in Hawaii. *Hawaii Journal of Medicine & Public Health, 71*(4 Suppl 1), 13–20.

American Hospital Association (2018). Fast facts on U.S. hospitals. www.aha.org/statistics/fast-facts-us-hospitals.

Associated Press (2018). Why care at Native American hospitals is often substandard. *The New York Times*, Section A, Pg. 4. https://www.nytimes.com/2016/10/09/us/why-care-at-native-american-hospitals-is-often-substandard.html

Becker, M. P., Collins, P. F., Schultz, A., Urošević, S., Schmaling, B., & Luciano, M. (2018). Longitudical changes in cognition in young adult cannabis users. *Journal of Clinical and Experimental Neuropsychology, 40*(6), 529–543. doi:10.1080/13803395.2017.1385-729

Braithwaite, L. F. (2016). Less Than 50% of teens identify as straight, says new study. Out. *News & Opinion.* https://www.out.com/news-opinion/2016/3/11/less-50-teens-identify-straight-says-new-study

Bratsberg, B., & Rogeberg, O. (2018). Flynn effect and its reversal are both environmentally caused. *Proceedings of the National Academy of Sciences of the United States of America, 115*(26), 6674–6678. doi:10.1073/pnas.1718793115

Centers for Disease Control and Prevention. Trends in the prevalence of marijuana, cocaine, and other illegal drug use, National YRBS: 1991–2017. https://www.cdc.gov/healthyyouth/data/yrbs/pdf/trends/2017_us_drug_trend_yrbs.pdf

Dockrill, P. (2018). IQ Scores are falling in "worrying" reversal of 20th Century intelligence boom. Science, *Alert*, https://www.sciencealert.com/iq-scores-falling-in-worrying-reversal-20th-century-intelligence-boom-flynn-effect-intelligence

Fitzsimons, T. (2018). A record 4.5 percent of U.S. adults identify as LGBT, Gallup Estimates. https://www.nbcnews.com/feature/nbc-out/record-4-5-percent-u-s-adults-identify-lgbt-gallup-n877486

Flores, A., Herman, J. L., Gates, G. J., & Brown, T. N. T. (2016). How many adults identify as transgender in the United States? Los Angeles, CA: The Williams Institute.

Gray, A. (2016). Where are all the Native doctors? *Association of American Indian Physicians*, https://www.aaip.org/media/news/m.blog/76/where-are-all-the-native-doctors

Hanes, S. (2015). Singles nation: Why so many Americans are unmarried. *The Christian Science Monitor*, https://www.csmonitor.com/USA/Society/2015/0614/Singles-nation-Why-so-many-Americans-are-unmarried

Johnson, M. (2018). The Healthcare future is female. *Athenahealth*, https://www.athenahealth.com/insight/healthcare-future-female

Kaiser Foundation (2018). Total number of professionally active nurses by gender. *The National Nursing Database*, https://www.kff.org/other/state-indicator/total-number-of-professionally-active-nurses-by-gender/?currentTimeframe=0&sortModel=%7B%22colId%22:%22Location%22,%22sort%22:%22asc%22%7D

Kane, C. K. (2015). Updated data on physician practice arrangements: Inching toward hospital ownership. *Policy Research Perspectives, American Medical Association*, http://www.ama-assn.org/resources/doc/health-policy/x-pub/prp-practice-arrangement-2015.pdf

Trustify, (2018). Infidelity statistics 2018: Why, when, and how people stray. www.trustify.info/blog/infidelity-statistics-2018

Glossary

A

Ableism The concept that people with "disabilities" are subjected to adverse attitudes, beliefs, and behaviors that generate feelings of inferiority and/or superiority.

Achieved Power Accomplishments that accrue through self-effort rather than by birth are defined as occurring through achieved power. (Conversely, accomplishments that accompany birth are referred to as ascribed power.)

Ageism Preconceived adverse attitudes, beliefs, and behaviors that result in feelings of inferiority and/or superiority based upon age.

C

Cultural Diversitisms Adverse attitudes, beliefs, and behaviors that are directed toward one group by another based on differences in the "way of life."

Cortisol This is a stress hormone that is produced in the adrenal glands.

D

DHEA (Dehydroepiandrosterone) This term references a naturally produced steroid hormone that is produced in the brain, the adrenal glands, and the sexual organs.

Disinhibition A behavioral process that is generated by power acquisition. It causes individuals to feel detached from existing social folkways and mores and prompts them to act on their individual impulses instead.

Dispersion The total and/or average degree to which a set of variables differ from the mean.

Diversitism All beliefs, attitudes, and actions, whether positive or negative, that are based upon human differences.

Diversity Dimensions This term refers to a de-identified analysis of the number and percent of people in the workplace who hold membership in various subgroups that experience incivilities because of their characteristics.

E

Edutainment An effective strategy that demonstrates the need for change through various modes of entertainment. Edutainment generates the introspection that is a necessary prerequisite to behavioral change.

EEOC The Equal Employment Opportunity Commission (EEOC) is responsible for enforcing federal laws that make it illegal to discriminate against a job applicant or an employee because of the person's race, color, religion, sex (including pregnancy, gender identity, and sexual orientation), national origin, age (40 or older), disability, or genetic information.

Eve teasing Sexual harassment acts that take place in mainly public places. Usually harassment of strangers who are predominately young girls and women.

External Directives Directives on discrimination that are assigned to the labor attorney and the labor economist of the Equal Employment Opportunity Commission for review and analysis.

H

Heterosexism A system of values and beliefs that views people who engage in same-sex or multi-sex relationships as inferior to individuals who are considered heterosexual.

I

Incivility Negative treatment by any human towards another human or other conscious living organism.

Intervention An action taken by one party so that a change in the course or an improvement of a condition or situation can occur in the awareness and actions of the second party.

Investigational Directives Related directives that guide the collection of evidence to support an EEOC claim.

IQism A system that rank orders individuals and defines them as inferior and/or superior based on perceptions of the individual's cognitive skills. Cognitive skills can be defined as an individual's ability to use thinking and reasoning skills.

Isms A distinctive doctrine, cause, or theory that leads to beliefs regarding the inferiority and/or superiority of one living thing versus another.

L

Linguicism Patterns of beliefs, attitudes, and behaviors that devalue others and reduce their professional and/or personal opportunities because of language.

Lookism A set of beliefs, attitudes, and behaviors that devalue or elevate others based on physical appearance.

M

Macro-level The term "macro" is a derivative of the Greek word Makros, which means "large." Thus, it can be argued that change is needed at the level of the society as a whole.

Mean The arithmetic mean refers to the value obtained when all numerical representations of some aspect of reality are first summed and then divided by the number of values in that universe of interest. This number, which is a quantitative average of all values, then *represents* the other values.

Micro-aggression Unconscious statements or actions that demean or insult another individual based on his or her group or subgroup membership.

Micro-assault Actions that are overt phenomena of subgroup discrimination. It may involve the use of harsh words and language or other intentional acts.

Micro-insult Negative statements regarding an individual's subgroup.

Micro-invalidation Behaviors and/or statements that dismiss the thoughts, feelings, and/or beliefs of an individual from another subgroup.

Micro-level Micro-level refers to change at the level of the individual person and/or other entity.

Multiple Intelligences Bodily, verbal-linguistic, logical-mathematical, musical, naturalistic, visual-spatial, and intrapersonal "gifts" that exceed the mean for humans as a collective. "Cognitively gifted" individuals have an advantage in verbal-linguistic and logical-mathematical skills.

N

Nameism The concept that a name can lead to implicit bias.

Nonverbal Communications Gestures, facial expressions, tone of voice, eye contact (or lack thereof), body language, posture, and other ways people can communicate without using language.

Normatively The act of viewing human behaviors as "good" or "bad" based on the ethics of a group. (In contrast, positive science is based upon measurable characteristics.)

O

Output Maximization The production of the largest amount and highest quality of output possible from available human and nonhuman resources.

P

Propinquity The state of being physically close to someone or something; "proximity" (technical sense); "close kinship."

Q

Quid pro quo Latin term that translates to "something for something."

R

Reinforcement Theory The theory that behaviors can be influenced by directly following desirable behaviors with rewards and by attaching negative consequences to undesirable behavior.

S

Sectarianism Fractured religious and/or other groups with their own strongly held beliefs, attitudes, and behaviors.

Self-Determination Theory (SDT) The belief that forces internal to individuals often drive their behavioral choices.

Sexism Prejudice or discrimination based on sex (especially discrimination against women).

Sexual assault Any behavior in which one individual touches another individual's body, including genitals, breasts, buttocks, lips, and/or other body parts for the purposes of sexual arousement and/or sexual pleasure without stated consent.

Sexual harassment All unwelcome actions that are of a sexual nature, i.e., catcalls, other inappropriate verbal speech, repeated sexual overtures, sexual advances, quid pro quo proposals, or other verbal or physical conduct of an unwelcome sexual nature.

Sexual Orientation A person's sexual identity in relation to the gender to which they are attracted; the fact of being heterosexual, homosexual, or bisexual.

Sexualism The innate desire for sex or sexuality in general that accompanies all members of the animal kingdom.

Somatization The conversion of a mental state (such as depression or anxiety) into physical symptoms. Somatization is often a factor in the aftermath of sexual harassment and/or sexual assault.

Structural unemployment The presence and availability of jobs in the workplace. However, there is a mismatch between the available jobs and the skills of the workers in search of employment.

T

Tendency An inclination toward particular characteristics or types of behaviors.

Theory of Central Tendencyism A framework for understanding the emergence and operation of the various systems of adverse beliefs, attitudes, and behaviors that assigns differential value to healthcare and other workers based upon the degree to which they differ from the mean or some other measure of that which a group considers as "normal."

Training Organized activity aimed at imparting information and/or instruction to improve the recipient's performance or to help him or her obtain a required level of knowledge or skill.

Transactional Sex Behaviors in which two individuals do not engage in sexual activity based on the reading of signals. Rather, a process of barter for material, financial, and/or other gain occurs as the "price" of sexual access.

Triarchic Theory Divides human intelligence into practical skills and the strengths associated with the introduction of other types of original approaches.

U

Uncivil Not civilized, barbarous, lacking in courtesy, ill-mannered, impolite, uncivil remarks, not conducive to civil harmony and welfare.

Unconstrained inclusion We introduce the term "unconstrained inclusion" to reference workplaces that include minimal levels of "Isms" that may reduce and/or limit output maximization.

Underdeveloped Humanisms Any and all attitudes, beliefs, and behaviors directed toward others that have a negative effect on that individual.

W

Workplace Isms A set of negative beliefs, values, attitudes, and behaviors by one subgroup regarding another. These beliefs, values, attitudes and behaviors undermine productivity in workplaces. These "Isms" may include but are not limited to variables such as ageism, racism, sexism, and others.

Index